# BEATING BACK PAIN

# 7 Natural Secrets for Lasting Relief

Second Edition

Dr. Joseph Jacobs, DPT, ACN

Second Edition, January 2026

Published by ASTR Institute
614 E HWY 50 #169, Clermont, FL 34711

ASTR

ASTRinstitute.com

# Disclaimer

This book, authored by Dr. Joseph Jacobs and published by the ASTR Institute, is intended for informational purposes only and presents medical research findings. It is not a substitute for professional medical advice, diagnosis, or treatment. Dr. Joseph Jacobs, the ASTR Institute, and its affiliates do not endorse or assume responsibility for any specific medical treatments or procedures discussed in this book. We strongly advise readers to consult with their healthcare providers regarding the applicability of any aspects of the content to their own health and well-being.

The statements contained herein have not been evaluated by the Food and Drug Administration. The products mentioned are not designed to diagnose, cure, treat, or prevent any disease. Individual results may vary, and we cannot guarantee that you will achieve the same outcomes as those detailed in our case studies, testimonials, and treatment videos. Success varies per individual, and one person's results do not guarantee similar outcomes for another.

If you have medical concerns, consult with your healthcare provider, physician, or another qualified medical professional. Dr. Joseph Jacobs, the ASTR Institute, and their associated organizations and individuals disclaim any liability for actions, services, or products acquired through this book, our videos, website, or any of our media channels.

# Table of Contents

# Online Resources

## How to Access Online Resources

Throughout this book, you'll find barcodes that link to additional online resources. Here's how to use them:

1. Open the camera app on your smartphone.
2. Point the camera at the barcode.
3. A notification will appear with a link. Tap the notification to open the link in your browser.

Triumph Over Trials: My Journey from Disability to Victory

After my second cancer treatment, I was suffering from chronic fatigue, migraines, muscle and joint pain. I reached out to at least seven doctors, but I could not find relief. Unfortunately, they had two responses. First, they said my blood labs looked normal. I learned from my studies in nutrition that this happened because they did not order the correct labs to figure out the root cause of my issues. The second response was that I was a hopeless case. This made me realize that if I wanted to overcome my disability, I had to look for a solution on my own. It was a difficult time in my life. Due to my pain and fatigue, it used to take me 10 minutes just to walk from the living room to the bathroom, about 20 feet away. I was very depressed and angry because, at 30 years old, I was facing numerous health issues and had a poor quality of life without any answers.

I spent countless hours and years studying nutrition, psychology, behavioral modification, anatomy, physiology, ergonomics, and other medical topics in hopes of finding an answer. At the same time, I was frustrated that the techniques I learned in medical school only provided short-term results with no lasting relief. I tried what I learned in school, such as stretching, exercises, electrical stimulation, various massage techniques, manual therapy, joint mobilization, and myofascial release, but nothing provided long-term results. So, I started to look at medical studies to guide me through this process. After reviewing over 16,000 medical research papers with assistance from medical students, I was shocked and disappointed by the results. Based on these studies, the following treatments either provided no pain reduction or only short-term pain reduction:

- NSAIDs
- Opioids
- Cortisone shots
- Exercises
- Stretching
- Massage
- Joint mobilization or manipulation
- Acupuncture
- Dry needling
- Instrument-assisted soft tissue mobilization

I have dedicated my life to researching all current traditional medical approaches to treating pain. I've found that the majority of these approaches primarily focus on relieving symptoms rather than addressing the root cause of the pain. The techniques I learned in school, still used in today's modern medical world, have their origins in ancient healing practices such as manipulation, massage, stretching, and exercise. These methods were used by the Romans, Greeks, and Egyptians to increase flexibility, strengthen muscles, and alleviate pain. Today's medicine has added treatments like cold, heat, electrical stimulation, and joint adjustment to this list. However, overwhelming evidence from published medical studies shows no promising long-term relief from any of these methods.

For instance, one systematic review conducted by the University of Ottawa, Canada, which reviewed 270 research studies, concluded that the benefits of massage, acupuncture, and spine adjustment treatments were mostly evident immediately or shortly after treatment, then faded over time. With compelling data like this, it is perplexing how we continue to treat patients with modalities that do not effectively address their long-term needs. Instead of focusing so much on the body's symptoms, we need to start questioning why these symptoms are present in the first place and why they keep returning.

This question guided me through an intense investigative research process over five years. From this research, I concluded that there are seven aspects of chronic pain that, when treated simultaneously, can lead to long-term pain relief. In my book, **Pain No More**, I outline seven key elements that must be addressed simultaneously to effectively relieve chronic pain. I also found that the BioPsychosocial model is an effective treatment approach for long-term pain reduction. So, I studied the BioPsychosocial model in depth and realized that my medical education was lacking in nutrition knowledge. I spent thousands of hours reading and studying nutrition and bought any book that I felt could help me understand the body better.

During this time, my wife had chronic jaw pain due to stress at work. I tried everything I learned from school on her, but nothing provided long-term pain relief. One day she woke up with lockjaw, unable to speak or open her mouth. She asked me to try anything. I told her that I had tried everything I knew, but nothing worked. So, I reached inside her mouth and experimented with several maneuvers. After a few minutes, she was able to open her mouth and was pain-free. I was dumbfounded and had no idea what had just happened. It took me several days to understand the physiology of the maneuvers I had performed. I then started experimenting with the same concept, applying it to the whole body to relieve both my pain and my patients' pain.

After several months of using my hands to implement the new maneuvers I had come up with, I realized I could not do that long-term. My hands were very sore, and I suffered from pain every night. I told my wife that this was not sustainable because I was in so much pain from using my hands. While patients were getting relief, I was suffering. My wife suggested that I use tools instead of my hands. So, I went to a hardware store and bought rubber, plastic, and metal to cut and design tools and devices to replace my hand maneuvers. Thankfully, this provided even faster results for my patients without me feeling soreness from working on them.

I was able to overcome my chronic fatigue and migraines by running comprehensive lab tests. These tests revealed several vitamin, mineral, and hormonal imbalances. Additionally, I overcame my chronic joint and muscle pain through the biopsychosocial (BPS) model and the tools and devices I invented. I also reinvented the biopsychosocial model to be implemented by a single healthcare provider and called it ASTR treatment.

My journey toward developing the ASTR diet was driven by personal challenges and professional insights. I experienced significant frustration with various diets that often left me feeling fatigued and unsatisfied. Through an extensive review of research studies, I also uncovered potential health risks associated with extreme dietary approaches. These experiences inspired me to create the ASTR Diet as a healthier, evidence-based alternative, which I share in my book **Eat to Heal**.

For years, I suffered from debilitating migraines and back pain, searching for lasting relief beyond temporary fixes. My journey as both a patient and a healthcare provider led me to dedicate 15 years to researching, studying, and testing effective solutions. Through this process, I developed a comprehensive approach that transformed my own health and has helped countless patients overcome chronic migraines and back pain. In this book, I share these evidence-based strategies, solutions that I have refined through experience and clinical practice. My hope is that this book serves as a practical guide to empower you on your path to recovery, providing the tools and knowledge needed to reclaim a pain-free life.

The Roadmap to Healing

**The Roadmap to Healing: A Comprehensive Approach to Beating Back Pain**

Back pain is one of the most complex and misunderstood conditions, often presenting as more than just discomfort or stiffness. It is a systemic issue, influenced by multiple underlying factors that can vary from person to person. Through 15 years of research, clinical practice, and personal experience, I have found that back pain is rarely triggered by a single element. Instead, it is the result of a combination of factors such as inflammatory food, poor posture, poor body mechanics, chronic stress, hormonal imbalances, environmental toxins, and deficiencies in essential vitamins and minerals. It is common to find that individuals suffering from back pain have at least five to seven contributing triggers, making an individualized and holistic approach to treatment essential for lasting relief.

In this chapter, I introduce a structured roadmap to healing, seven natural secrets to lasting relief, designed to address the root causes of back pain rather than just suppressing symptoms. **These elements are interconnected, and for the best results, it is crucial to implement all seven.** Each component plays a key role in restoring balance to the body, reducing inflammation, and optimizing musculoskeletal and nervous system function. When one or more of these factors are overlooked, back pain often persists or returns, which is why a comprehensive approach is necessary.

By following this roadmap, you are not just managing your back pain; you are taking control of your health and actively working toward eliminating it at its source. **This method is not about quick fixes or temporary relief; it's about equipping your body with the tools it needs to heal naturally and sustainably.** With dedication and consistency, you can break free from chronic back pain and regain your quality of life, just as I did and as my patients have done.

**Case Studies**

This chapter presents real-life case studies of individuals who have successfully implemented the ASTR approach to overcome chronic back pain. Each case study highlights the patient's unique challenges, treatment strategies, and outcomes. These stories provide valuable insights and inspiration for readers, demonstrating the effectiveness of a holistic, science-based approach to back pain relief. This chapter includes a QR code to watch these case studies.

**Understanding Back Pain**

This chapter provides a comprehensive exploration of back pain, including its neurological and physiological mechanisms. It delves into the role of the musculoskeletal system, nerve compression, inflammatory responses, postural imbalances, and genetic predispositions. Readers will gain a deeper understanding of how back pain develops, the various types of back pain, and the factors that contribute to its frequency and severity. This chapter lays the foundation for the holistic approach to back pain relief presented in the book.

**Navigating the Healing Journey: How Your Body Recovers Naturally**

This chapter explores the normal body healing cycle, detailing the intricate processes that allow the body to repair and recover naturally. It explains how the immune system, nervous system, and cellular mechanisms work together to promote healing, reduce inflammation, and restore balance. In contrast, the chapter also examines the chronic back pain cycle, highlighting the internal disruptions that prevent proper healing. Chronic back pain often results from a combination of musculoskeletal dysfunction, heightened pain sensitivity, inflammation, and metabolic imbalances, leading to recurring and persistent discomfort. By understanding the differences between the body's natural healing response and the back pain cycle, readers will gain valuable insights. This knowledge empowers them to break free from the repetitive nature of chronic back pain and effectively support their body's ability to heal.

**7 Natural Secrets**

**1. Inflammatory Foods**

Certain foods can contribute to back pain by triggering inflammatory responses, disrupting muscle function, or affecting nerve health. This chapter outlines the most common back pain-triggering foods, including processed sugars, artificial additives, and inflammatory fats. It introduces the ASTR Diet's approach to help readers identify their personal triggers and transition to a back pain-friendly, nutrient-dense diet.

## 2. Imbalance: Vitamins, Minerals, and Hormones

Nutritional deficiencies and hormonal imbalances play a critical role in back pain frequency and severity. This chapter discusses how deficiencies in magnesium, vitamin D, B vitamins, and other essential nutrients contribute to muscle tension, inflammation, and nerve dysfunction. It also explores how hormonal fluctuations, particularly estrogen, cortisol, and thyroid hormones, affect pain sensitivity and musculoskeletal health. Practical strategies for restoring balance through diet, supplementation, and lifestyle modifications are provided.

## 3. Posture

Poor posture, especially in the spine, is a significant but often overlooked contributor to back pain. This chapter examines how misalignments in the neck, shoulders, and lower back can lead to muscle tension, nerve compression, and reduced mobility. Readers will learn about postural correction techniques, ergonomic adjustments, and exercises that can alleviate back pain symptoms and prevent recurrence.

## 4. Stress Management

Chronic stress is a major contributor to back pain, as it leads to hormonal imbalances, muscle tension, and heightened nervous system sensitivity. This chapter introduces effective stress management techniques, including mindfulness, deep breathing exercises, and relaxation strategies. It also discusses how emotional health and unresolved trauma can impact pain levels and provides practical steps for fostering mental and emotional resilience.

## 5. Fibrotic Tissue

Scar tissue and fibrotic adhesions can develop in response to injuries, chronic inflammation, or repetitive strain, leading to muscle tightness and restricted movement. This chapter explores how fibrotic tissue in the back and surrounding muscles can contribute to chronic pain by impairing circulation, nerve function, and mobility.

## 6. Fascial Restriction

The fascia, a connective tissue network that surrounds muscles and organs, plays a crucial role in movement and pain regulation. When the fascia becomes restricted, it can lead to tension and discomfort, including chronic back pain. This chapter explains the connection between fascial restrictions and musculoskeletal dysfunction and introduces methods for restoring fascial health.

## 7. Behavior Modification

Long-term back pain relief requires lasting changes in lifestyle habits and behaviors. This chapter examines the impact of sleep patterns, hydration, physical activity, and environmental factors on pain prevention. It provides guidance on habit formation, self-monitoring techniques, and strategies for sustaining positive lifestyle changes to ensure lasting relief from back pain.

Case Studies & Research

All case studies presented in this book illustrate that a holistic approach to back pain treatment can be effectively implemented by a single healthcare provider. A holistic approach considers the interconnected systems of the body, addressing not only the symptoms of back pain but also the underlying causes that contribute to its recurrence. This method integrates multiple elements, including nutritional balance, musculoskeletal health, stress management, lifestyle adjustments, and behavioral modifications, to create a comprehensive treatment plan tailored to the individual's needs.

By focusing on the root causes rather than just symptom management, a holistic approach can identify and correct deficiencies in vitamins, minerals, and hormones. It also addresses postural imbalances, reduces fibrotic tissue and fascial restrictions, and implements behavior modification techniques to support long-term healing. This integrative method not only helps in alleviating pain but also promotes long-term wellness and prevention of future back pain episodes.

The case studies and recorded live treatment videos available online provide real-life examples of how this approach is applied in practice. To watch these case studies and treatment videos, use the barcode provided in this book or visit the following link:

https://advancedsofttissuerelease.com/treatment-videos-2/

## Case Study 1: 8 Years of Neck Pain

**Diagnosis:** Neck disc herniation from car accident
**Symptoms:** Sharp neck pain, right arm/shoulder dull aching pain, limited range of motion, and limited activities.

**Previous Failed Treatments:** Physical therapy and trigger point injection.
**Length of Injury:** 8 years.
**Pain Level on a Scale of 0 to 10:** 6-8/10.
**Treatment:** Treatment included releasing fibrotic tissue, addressing fascia restrictions, decreasing inflammation, improving ergonomics, implementing an anti-inflammatory diet, and addressing vitamin, mineral, and hormonal imbalances.
**Outcome:** Symptoms resolved.

## Case Study 2: 1 Month of Neck Pain

**Diagnosis:** Neck pain after workout.
**Symptoms:** Constant dull/sharp neck and upper back pain
**Previous Failed Treatments:** Foam roller.
**Length of Injury:** 1 month.
**Pain Level on a Scale of 0 to 10:** 3-9/10.
**Treatment:** Treatment included releasing fibrotic tissue, addressing fascia restrictions, decreasing inflammation, improving ergonomics, and implementing an anti-inflammatory diet.
**Outcome:** Symptoms resolved.

## Case Study 3: 16 Years of Neck Pain

**Diagnosis:** Neck pain after car accident.
**Symptoms:** Neck and traps pain.
**Previous Failed Treatments:** Chiropractor, massage therapy, and physical therapy.
**Length of Injury:** 16 years.
**Pain Level on a Scale of 0 to 10:** 6-7/10.
**Treatment:** Treatment included releasing fibrotic tissue, addressing fascia restrictions, decreasing inflammation, improving ergonomics, and implementing an anti-inflammatory diet.
**Outcome:** Symptoms resolved.

## Case Study 4: 10 Years of Neck and Shoulder Pain

**Diagnosis:** Neck and shoulder pain after car accident.
**Symptoms:** Neck pain, trapezius pain, muscle spasm, difficulty driving, difficulty sleeping, and limited shoulder flexion.
**Previous Failed Treatments:** 6 different physical therapists, 2 different chiropractors, and acupuncture.
**Length of Injury:** 10 years.
**Pain Level on a Scale of 0 to 10:** 3-10/10.
**Treatment:** Treatment included releasing fibrotic tissue, addressing fascia restrictions, decreasing inflammation, improving ergonomics, and implementing an anti-inflammatory diet.
**Outcome:** Symptoms resolved.

## Case Study 5: 30 Years of Back Pain and Bilateral Leg Numbness

**Diagnosis:** Back pain after lifting a wheelchair.
**Symptoms:** Constant back pain, aching and stabbing, with radiation to bilateral lower extremities, tingling, and numbness, limping stiff gait, and unable to sleep on bed.
**Previous Failed Treatments:** Back fusion surgery and physical therapy.
**Length of Injury:** 30 years.
**Pain Level on a Scale of 0 to 10:** 3-10/10.
**Treatment:** Treatment included releasing fibrotic tissue, addressing fascia restrictions, decreasing inflammation, improving ergonomics, implementing an anti-inflammatory diet, and addressing vitamin, mineral, and hormonal imbalances.
**Outcome:** Symptoms resolved.

## Case Study 6: 7 Years of Back Pain and Leg Pain

**Diagnosis:** Back pain after car accidents.
**Symptoms:** Constant back pain, thigh/ leg pain, unable to sit up on bed, and very stiff back.
**Previous Failed Treatments:** back ablation surgery, a lot physical therapy, and a lot of massage therapy.
**Length of Injury:** 7 years.
**Pain Level on a Scale of 0 to 10:** 3-10/10.
**Treatment:** Treatment included releasing fibrotic tissue, addressing fascia

restrictions, decreasing inflammation, improving ergonomics, implementing an anti-inflammatory diet.
**Outcome:** Symptoms resolved.

## Case Study 7: 2 Years of Low Back Pain

**Diagnosis:** Low back pain.
**Symptoms:** Low back pain, muscle spasm, and numbness/ needle pain.
**Previous Failed Treatments:**
**Length of Injury:** 2 years.
**Pain Level on a Scale of 0 to 10:** 7-9/10.
**Treatment:** Treatment included releasing fibrotic tissue, addressing fascia restrictions, decreasing inflammation, improving ergonomics, implementing an anti-inflammatory diet.
**Outcome:** Symptoms resolved.

Feel free to scan the QR code below to watch more live treatment cases.

## Research Evidence

Back pain is not a single-cause condition. It is one of the most common and costly chronic health problems worldwide, and it often becomes persistent because multiple systems are involved at the same time. Pain sensitivity, inflammation, tissue healing, posture and movement mechanics, nervous system stress responses, sleep, nutrition, fascia, scar tissue behavior, and daily habits can all shape whether back pain resolves quickly or becomes chronic. Modern research increasingly supports one major conclusion: lasting recovery requires a whole-person framework, not a single intervention or a single diagnosis.

This book is grounded in the **biopsychosocial model**, a scientific framework introduced by George Engel to address the limitations of viewing chronic illness as only a mechanical or structural problem (Engel, 1977). The biopsychosocial model recognizes that back pain is driven by three interacting domains:

- **Biological factors**, including inflammation, oxidative stress, nutrient status, hormonal regulation, connective tissue remodeling, nerve sensitivity, and tissue fibrosis
- **Psychological factors**, including stress physiology, fear, pain-related beliefs, trauma load, emotional regulation, and nervous system reactivity
- **Social and behavioral factors**, including movement habits, posture demands, sedentary patterns, sleep routines, work stress, and long-term consistency of lifestyle behaviors

This model is not a "soft" theory. It is supported by decades of clinical and epidemiological research showing that chronic pain outcomes are shaped by systems interacting in real time, rather than a single damaged structure (Borrell-Carrió et al., 2004).

## The Biomedical Model: Strengths and Limitations

Conventional back pain care is still largely built on the biomedical model, which assumes pain is caused primarily by structural injury or tissue damage that can be identified, isolated, and corrected. In this framework, back pain is often reduced to findings such as disc degeneration, bulging discs, arthritis, spinal alignment changes, or muscle strain. The biomedical model has real strengths. It helps identify red flags such as fracture, infection, tumor, severe neurological compromise, or inflammatory spinal disease. It also supports appropriate acute care, imaging when clinically justified, and targeted interventions when a clear structural cause is present.

However, its limitation is scope. Many people suffer persistent back pain without a proportional structural explanation. Large imaging studies show that "degenerative" spine findings are common even in pain-free people, and these findings increase with age (Brinjikji et al., 2015). This means imaging abnormalities can be present without being the true driver of symptoms. The biomedical approach often treats the back like a broken part, rather than a living system influenced by inflammation, fascia mobility, stress hormones, movement patterns, nutrient status, sleep, and behavioral reinforcement loops. This is one reason so many patients experience recurring episodes, persistent pain, treatment fatigue, and chronic disability despite "normal" test results or repeated symptom-based therapies.

**The Biopsychosocial Model: A Systems-Based Framework for Back Pain**

## Biopsychosocial

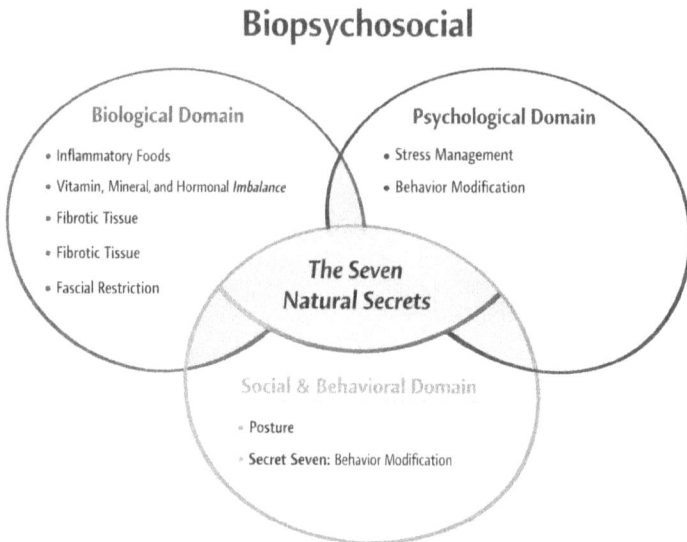

**Biological Domain**
- Inflammatory Foods
- Vitamin, Mineral, and Hormonal *Imbalance*
- Fibrotic Tissue
- Fibrotic Tissue
- Fascial Restriction

**Psychological Domain**
- Stress Management
- Behavior Modification

*The Seven Natural Secrets*

Social & Behavioral Domain
- Posture
- **Secret Seven:** Behavior Modification

The biopsychosocial model explains why back pain is often persistent even when imaging does not show severe injury. It reframes pain as a biological output shaped by multiple interacting inputs. This model aligns with large-scale research describing back pain as a complex condition influenced by tissue health, nervous system sensitivity, behavior patterns, psychological load, and environmental pressure (Hartvigsen et al., 2018).

The **seven natural secrets** in this book are organized directly around that biopsychosocial structure. Each secret reflects one or more domains of the model:

**Biological domain**

Secret One: Inflammatory Foods
Secret Two: Vitamin, Mineral, and Hormonal Imbalance
Secret Five: Fibrotic Tissue
Secret Six: Fascial Restriction

**Psychological domain**
Secret Four: Stress Management
Secret Seven: Behavior Modification

**Social and Behavioral domain**
Secret Three: Posture
Secret Seven: Behavior Modification

This chapter presents the scientific evidence supporting each category. Practical strategies and implementation are reserved for the chapters that follow.

# Biopsychosocial

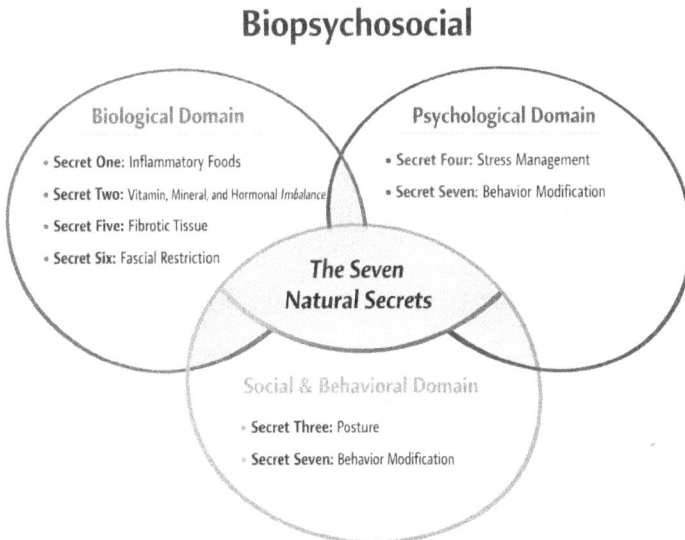

**Biological Domain**
• **Secret One:** Inflammatory Foods
• **Secret Two:** Vitamin, Mineral, and Hormonal Imbalance
• **Secret Five:** Fibrotic Tissue
• **Secret Six:** Fascial Restriction

**Psychological Domain**
• **Secret Four:** Stress Management
• **Secret Seven:** Behavior Modification

*The Seven Natural Secrets*

**Social & Behavioral Domain**
• **Secret Three:** Posture
• **Secret Seven:** Behavior Modification

**Secret One: Inflammatory Foods**

**Evidence that diet-driven inflammation is linked to pain persistence**

Chronic back pain is not only mechanical. A growing body of research shows that systemic inflammation can amplify pain sensitivity, disrupt tissue recovery, and worsen musculoskeletal symptoms. Diet is a major driver of inflammation because it shapes blood sugar stability, oxidative stress load, gut-derived inflammatory signaling, and immune activation. Large reviews consistently associate high intake of ultra-processed foods with worse cardiometabolic outcomes and chronic inflammatory patterns (Lane et al., 2024). These inflammatory pathways are increasingly linked to chronic pain vulnerability. Diet quality also influences pain through the concept of dietary inflammatory potential. Higher Dietary Inflammatory Index scores have been associated with chronic pain outcomes in population-based studies, supporting the broader inflammatory connection between food patterns and persistent pain states (Qing et al., 2024).

This evidence aligns with mechanistic research showing that inflammatory dietary patterns can increase cytokine signaling, impair mitochondrial energy production, and contribute to pain sensitization pathways over time. In the biopsychosocial model, inflammatory foods act as a biological driver that is reinforced by lifestyle patterns and behavioral repetition.

**Secret Two: Vitamin, Mineral, and Hormonal Imbalance**

**Evidence that physiology and endocrine regulation influence back pain outcomes**

Back pain recovery depends on healthy nerve signaling, muscle function, connective tissue remodeling, and anti-inflammatory regulation. These processes rely heavily on micronutrient sufficiency and hormone balance. Research consistently shows that nutrient deficiencies can worsen pain sensitivity, impair healing, and reduce functional recovery. Vitamin D, for example, has been widely studied in chronic pain because it supports immune regulation, muscle performance, and inflammatory control. Although findings vary by population and baseline deficiency status, randomized trials and meta-analyses continue to evaluate vitamin D's role in chronic low back pain outcomes (Ghai et al., 2017; Lee et al., 2024).

Hormonal regulation is also relevant because hormones shape inflammation, tissue repair, sleep quality, mood stability, and muscle tension thresholds.,Cortisol disruption, thyroid imbalance, insulin resistance, and sex hormone instability can each alter inflammatory tone and pain processing, making pain more persistent and less responsive to isolated interventions.

In the biopsychosocial model, vitamin, mineral, and hormonal imbalances represent a biological vulnerability layer. When this layer is ignored, pain may continue even when posture work, stretching, or symptom management is attempted.

**Secret Three: Posture**

**Evidence that mechanical load and sustained positions shape pain risk**

Posture is not simply about looking aligned. It is about how the spine is loaded repeatedly, how long the same tissues stay under tension, and how movement variability is reduced over time. Occupational research has consistently shown that back pain risk increases when posture demands combine with other stressors such as vibration exposure, prolonged static positions, and awkward mechanics. A major review found that prolonged sitting alone is not always sufficient to cause pain, but sitting combined with vibration and awkward posture significantly increases low back pain risk (Lis et al., 2006).

Sedentary behavior has also been associated with increased low back pain risk across adult and youth populations. A systematic review reported that sedentary behavior, whether at work or during leisure time, is linked to a moderate increase in low back pain risk (Mahdavi et al., 2021). This matters because the spine adapts to repeated patterns. When posture habits reduce spinal movement diversity, the nervous system may begin to interpret normal loading as threatening, increasing protective muscle tension and pain signals. Within the biopsychosocial model, posture is both a biological load factor and a behavioral repetition factor, shaped by routine, work environment, and daily habits.

**Secret Four: Stress Management**

**Evidence that stress physiology can intensify pain and disability**

Stress is not just emotional. It is physiological. Chronic stress activates the sympathetic nervous system and the hypothalamic-pituitary-adrenal axis, increasing cortisol, adrenaline output, muscle guarding, inflammatory signaling, and sleep disruption. This stress-pain link is strongly supported in chronic low back pain research. A major randomized clinical trial found that mindfulness-based stress reduction improved functional outcomes and pain-related measures in chronic low back pain compared with usual care, with benefits persisting over time (Cherkin et al., 2016).

A growing body of evidence supports stress-based interventions because they reduce pain amplification, improve coping capacity, and decrease nervous system hypersensitivity. Psychological burden does not "cause" pain in the sense of imagining it. Instead, stress physiology can amplify pain processing, increase muscle tension, worsen inflammation, and reduce recovery bandwidth. Within the biopsychosocial model, stress management represents the psychological domain directly influencing biological pain output.

**Secret Five: Fibrotic Tissue**

**Evidence that scar-like remodeling and adhesions can contribute to persistent pain**

Fibrosis refers to excessive or abnormal connective tissue remodeling. In pain states, fibrosis can reduce tissue glide, increase mechanical stiffness, trap inflammatory signaling locally, and increase nerve irritation through adhesions or restricted movement of tissues.This is especially well documented in post-surgical spine pain. Postoperative epidural fibrosis is recognized as a common contributor to persistent pain after spine surgery and is a leading factor in failed back surgery syndrome (Lewik et al., 2023). Fibrotic change is also deeply linked to myofibroblast activity, which drives collagen deposition and tissue contracture. Fibrosis research identifies myofibroblasts as key effector cells in connective tissue stiffening and remodeling across multiple fibrotic conditions (Monument et al., 2015).

Even outside of surgery, fibrosis-like remodeling may contribute to chronic musculoskeletal pain patterns by reducing tissue adaptability and increasing mechanical resistance during normal movement. In the biopsychosocial model, fibrotic tissue represents a biological persistence factor that can maintain pain even after inflammation improves.

## Secret Six: Fascial Restriction

### Evidence that fascia mobility changes are measurable in chronic low back pain

Fascia is not passive wrapping. It is a living connective tissue network containing sensory receptors, collagen fibers, hydration layers, and mechanical force transmission properties. Research has shown measurable differences in fascia structure and movement in chronic low back pain: Langevin and colleagues found ultrasound evidence of altered lumbar connective tissue structure in people with chronic low back pain compared with controls (Langevin et al., 2009). Later work demonstrated reduced thoracolumbar fascia shear strain in chronic low back pain patients, supporting the concept that fascia movement quality can be impaired in persistent pain states (Langevin et al., 2011).

These findings matter because fascial restriction can contribute to pain by reducing normal tissue glide, increasing stiffness, altering movement mechanics, and feeding protective muscle guarding responses. Within the biopsychosocial model, fascia restriction is primarily a biological domain factor, but it is often reinforced by behavioral patterns such as immobility, repetitive movement, and postural rigidity.

## Secret Seven: Behavior Modification

### Evidence that beliefs, fear, habits, and consistency shape pain outcomes

One of the most research-supported contributors to chronic back pain is the role of behavioral reinforcement loops. Pain changes behavior. Then behavior changes the nervous system. Over time, this can lock pain into a persistent cycle. A classic model explaining this is the fear-avoidance framework, which describes how pain-related fear can lead to movement avoidance, physical deconditioning, increased disability, and ongoing pain sensitivity (Vlaeyen & Linton, 2000).

Behavioral and cognitive patterns also shape central sensitization. Reviews show that central sensitization, a state of amplified nervous system responsiveness, is associated with higher pain intensity, worse outcomes, and reduced quality of life in chronic low back pain (den Bandt et al., 2019).

This is why biopsychosocial rehabilitation models have repeatedly outperformed isolated treatments. A major systematic review found that multidisciplinary biopsychosocial rehabilitation improves long-term outcomes for chronic low back pain compared with usual care (Kamper et al., 2015). Exercise therapy itself is supported by strong evidence, but its long-term value is strongly tied to behavior consistency, adherence, and habit integration. A Cochrane review found moderate-certainty evidence that exercise improves pain outcomes in chronic low back pain compared with usual care or placebo (Hayden et al., 2021). In the biopsychosocial model, behavior modification is where the entire system becomes sustainable. It links biological change to psychological regulation and social routines.

## Conclusion: A Scientific Model, Not Opinion

The research presented in this chapter shows that chronic back pain is not simply a spine problem. It is a whole-system condition driven by interconnected biology, psychology, and behavior. Inflammatory food exposure, micronutrient and hormonal disruption, posture strain, stress physiology, fibrotic remodeling, fascial restriction, and behavior reinforcement loops all measurably influence pain outcomes. The biopsychosocial model provides the unifying framework that explains why single-intervention care often produces incomplete results, and why a systems-based approach is required for lasting recovery (Engel, 1977; Hartvigsen et al., 2018). The chapters that follow will translate this evidence into focused, step-by-step strategies for each of the seven natural secrets, building directly on the research foundation established here.

# Understanding Back Pain

Back pain is a pervasive health issue affecting a substantial portion of the global population. In 2019, approximately 39.0% of adults in the United States reported experiencing back pain within a three-month period, with prevalence increasing with age and higher rates observed among women and non-Hispanic white adults (National Center for Health Statistics, 2020). Globally, low back pain affected an estimated 619 million people in 2020, and this number is projected to rise to 843 million by 2050, primarily due to population growth and aging (World Health Organization [WHO], 2022). Notably, low back pain is the leading cause of disability worldwide, underscoring its significant impact on individuals and healthcare systems (Institute for Health Metrics and Evaluation, 2023).

Regardless of the type of back pain you experience, whether it is caused by a herniated disc, muscle strain, sciatica, arthritis, or postural dysfunction, effective treatment must focus on addressing the root cause rather than just managing symptoms. The only exception is fractures, which require immediate stabilization. **The key to resolving chronic back pain lies in understanding the body's natural healing cycle, as this is the fundamental process the body relies on for recovery.**

Since the body follows a structured program of inflammation, repair, and remodeling to heal injuries, it is essential to identify where it is stuck in this cycle. If the body remains in a prolonged inflammatory phase or fails to transition into proper tissue regeneration, the pain persists. Therefore, the most effective approach is not merely treating the structural label of the injury but rather assessing and facilitating the body's ability to move through the healing process.

Regardless of the label your healthcare provider gives your condition, whether it is caused by a herniated disc, muscle strain, sciatica, arthritis, or postural dysfunction, effective healing is possible. These diagnostic labels primarily indicate the location and nature of the tissue involved but do not inherently dictate the best course of treatment. True healing requires a comprehensive approach that restores normal function, reduces inflammation, and optimizes musculoskeletal health rather than relying solely on interventions targeting the injury site. By focusing on the body's ability to heal rather than just the name of the condition, long-term recovery becomes more attainable and sustainable.

In this chapter, I briefly introduce the normal healing cycle to establish its relationship with various back injuries. Understanding this process is essential for addressing the root cause of back pain rather than remaining stuck with diagnostic labels such as sciatica, herniated discs, or spinal stenosis. While these labels describe the location and nature of an injury, they do not inherently dictate the most effective treatment approach. The healing cycle consists of three primary phases: inflammation, proliferation, and maturation, which work together to repair and restore damaged tissues. If the body becomes stuck in any of these phases, chronic pain and dysfunction may persist, preventing full recovery.

The next chapter explores the healing cycle in greater detail, offering a comprehensive understanding of how to facilitate proper recovery and support the body's natural healing ability. By shifting the focus from symptom

## Normal Healing Cycle

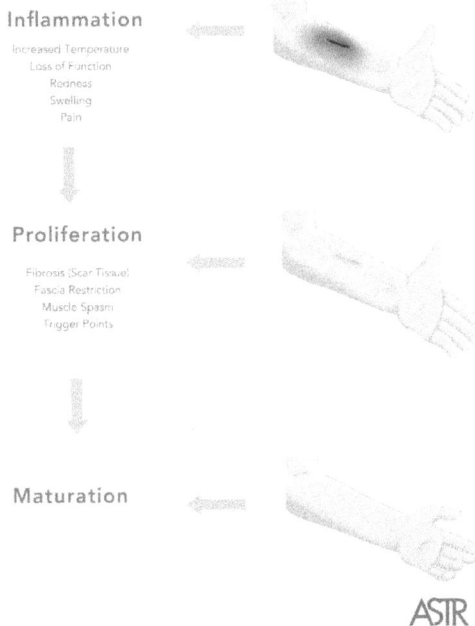

### Inflammation

Increased Temperature
Loss of Function
Redness
Swelling
Pain

### Proliferation

Fibrosis (Scar Tissue)
Fascia Restriction
Muscle Spasm
Trigger Points

### Maturation

ASTR

management to resolving dysfunction within the healing cycle, a more effective and long-lasting solution for back pain can be achieved.

**Normal Healing Cycle**

The normal healing cycle consists of three stages, which can be illustrated using an external paper cut to visualize what happens internally in the body. See the image above for more details. The first stage is inflammation, characterized by swelling, redness, pain, and increased blood flow to the affected area. The second stage involves the formation of fibrosis, also known as scar tissue, which fills the wound to prevent it from remaining open and susceptible to infection. During this stage, the injured site may also experience fascial restrictions and muscle spasms. This highlights the essential role of scar tissue in our protection and survival.

The third stage of the healing cycle involves the breakdown of fibrotic tissue. Ideally, in a perfect world with perfect bodies, the body would autonomously break down this fibrotic tissue over a period of days, weeks, or months, depending on the severity of the injury. However, we do not live in a perfect world. As we age, our body's ability to break down scar tissue decreases significantly.

This healing process also occurs internally when our bodies experience injuries from accidents, surgeries, trauma, poor posture, or stress. In chronic conditions, the injured area may not progress through all three stages, instead getting stuck between the inflammation and proliferation stages.

**Back Structures:**

The spine comprises several essential anatomical structures, each performing distinct and vital roles. **Vertebrae** are individual bones stacked vertically, forming the spinal column. They provide structural support, protect the spinal cord, and facilitate movements such as bending and twisting. Between these vertebrae lie the **intervertebral discs**, cushion-like structures composed of a fibrous outer ring (annulus fibrosus) and a gel-like inner core (nucleus pulposus). These discs absorb shock, evenly distribute pressure, and permit flexibility in spinal movements.

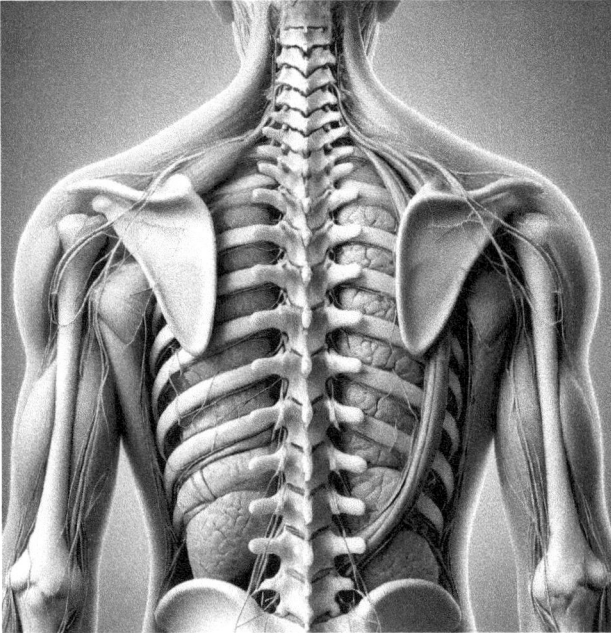

Running centrally through the vertebral column is the **spinal cord**, a critical bundle of nerve fibers extending from the brainstem downwards. From the spinal cord, **spinal nerves** branch outward through spaces between the vertebrae, serving as pathways for nerve signals that regulate movement, sensation, and autonomic bodily functions.

Surrounding and supporting these structures is the **fascia**, a connective tissue that envelops muscles, nerves, and other tissues. The fascia stabilizes anatomical components, reduces friction during movement, and distributes mechanical forces throughout the body.

Finally, muscles such as the **erector spinae group**, positioned parallel along the spine, significantly contribute to spinal health. These muscles maintain posture, stabilize the spinal column, and enable movements including extension, lateral flexion, and rotation. Together, these structures collaborate to ensure the spine's stability, flexibility, protective functions, and overall biomechanical effectiveness.

**Physiology of Back Pain**

The etiology of back pain is multifaceted, involving various anatomical structures such as muscles, ligaments, intervertebral discs, nerves, and vertebrae. Muscle strains or ligament sprains often result from overuse, improper lifting, or sudden movements, leading to acute pain (American Society of Anesthesiologists [ASA], 2023). Degeneration of intervertebral discs, a common aspect of aging, can diminish their cushioning ability, contributing to pain and reduced mobility. Herniated or ruptured discs occur when the soft nucleus of a disc protrudes through its outer layer, potentially compressing adjacent nerves and causing pain. Additionally, conditions like spinal stenosis, characterized by the narrowing of the spinal canal, can exert pressure on the spinal cord and nerves, leading to discomfort and neurological symptoms (National Institute of Neurological Disorders and Stroke [NINDS], 2020).

## Biomechanics of the Spine

The human spine is a complex structure comprising vertebrae, intervertebral discs, ligaments, and muscles, all working in unison to provide support, flexibility, and protection to the spinal cord. Biomechanical studies have shown that movements such as flexion, extension, rotation, and lateral flexion involve a combination of rotation and translation across different planes, resulting in various forces acting on the lumbar spine and sacrum. These forces include compression, shear, and tensile stresses, which, when excessive or improperly managed, can lead to tissue injury and pain.

## Types of Back Injuries and Their Relationship to the Healing Cycle

Back pain manifests in various forms, each with distinct characteristics and underlying causes. While these conditions may have different structural origins, their healing depends on the body's ability to progress through the normal healing cycle, which consists of three primary phases: inflammation, proliferation, and maturation. Understanding where the body is stuck within this process is essential for effective treatment and recovery.

## Sciatica

Sciatica results from compression or irritation of the sciatic nerve, often due to a herniated disc, fibrotic tissue in the piriformis muscle, or spinal stenosis. In the inflammatory phase, nerve irritation leads to pain, swelling, and dysfunction. If inflammation persists without resolution, the body struggles to transition to the proliferation phase, where damaged nerve tissues and surrounding structures begin healing.

## Herniated Disc

A herniated disc occurs when the nucleus of an intervertebral disc pushes through its outer layer, potentially compressing nearby nerves. The inflammatory phase is marked by pain, swelling, and nerve irritation. If left unresolved, chronic inflammation prevents the transition to the proliferation phase, where disc rehydration and healing should occur.

## Scoliosis

Scoliosis, an abnormal lateral curvature of the spine, causes chronic muscle imbalance and mechanical strain. While scoliosis itself may not "heal" in the traditional sense, managing its effects depends on supporting the maturation phase of the healing cycle. Since the body constantly adapts to postural stress, targeted therapy can guide structural changes, helping muscles and connective tissues function more efficiently despite the spinal misalignment.

## Osteoarthritis

Osteoarthritis of the spine results from cartilage deterioration in the facet joints, leading to pain, stiffness, and reduced flexibility. The inflammatory phase in osteoarthritis is often prolonged, causing chronic pain and joint degeneration. Effective treatment must focus on breaking the cycle of inflammation and facilitating the proliferation phase, where cartilage preservation strategies, such as proper nutrition, weight management, and anti-inflammatory therapies, support joint health. Exercise and mobility programs help strengthen surrounding muscles to support the maturation phase, improving movement patterns and reducing stress on affected joints.

## Spinal Stenosis

Spinal stenosis occurs when the spinal canal narrows, compressing the spinal cord and nerves. Chronic inflammation in stenotic regions leads to persistent pain and dysfunction, preventing the body from progressing through the healing cycle. Decompressive treatments, manual therapy, and exercises that reduce nerve compression help transition the body into the proliferation phase, allowing neural structures to function more efficiently. The maturation phase is supported through strength training and mobility exercises to enhance spinal stability and prevent further degeneration.

**Degenerative Disc Disease**

Degenerative disc disease results from gradual wear and tear of intervertebral discs, leading to reduced flexibility and chronic pain. If the body remains stuck in the inflammatory phase, ongoing pain and dysfunction prevent healing. Proper hydration, movement therapy, and targeted strengthening exercises facilitate the proliferation stage, allowing the body to stabilize weakened discs. In the remodeling phase, long-term postural adjustments and muscle reconditioning prevent further breakdown and support spine health.

**Spondylolisthesis**

Spondylolisthesis, where one vertebra slips forward over another, often causes nerve compression and back instability. Chronic inflammation surrounding the affected vertebra prevents healing, keeping the body in a prolonged inflammatory phase.

**Ankylosing Spondylitis**

Ankylosing spondylitis is an inflammatory arthritis that causes spinal stiffness and fusion over time. Because this condition is inflammatory in nature, the body is often trapped in the inflammatory phase, leading to ongoing pain and tissue damage. The goal of treatment is to regulate inflammation through diet, address vitamin and mineral deficiencies, and incorporate movement, allowing the body to enter the proliferation stage, where inflammation is controlled and symptoms are reduced. In the maturation phase, mobility exercises help prevent excessive spinal fusion and preserve function.

## Myofascial Pain Syndrome

Myofascial pain syndrome results from muscle overuse, stress, or injury, leading to localized pain and tightness in the fascia. Chronic tension prevents the body from transitioning beyond the inflammatory phase, causing persistent pain and dysfunction.

## Compression Fractures

Compression fractures, common in individuals with osteoporosis, occur when weakened vertebrae collapse, causing severe back pain. Unlike other conditions, fractures require immediate stabilization and structural support. The inflammatory phase involves pain and swelling, and treatment must prioritize immobilization and bone healing. The proliferation stage is supported through bone-strengthening interventions such as proper nutrition (calcium and vitamin D), medical management, and controlled movement therapy. In the maturation phase, weight-bearing exercises and postural adjustments help rebuild bone density and prevent future fractures.

## Failed Back Surgery Syndrome

Failed back surgery syndrome (FBSS) is a condition characterized by persistent or recurrent pain following spinal surgery, indicating that the procedure did not achieve the desired outcome. Despite advances in spinal surgery techniques, a significant proportion of patients continue to experience chronic pain after undergoing procedures intended to relieve their symptoms. FBSS is not a specific diagnosis but rather an umbrella term encompassing various causes of post-surgical pain, including inadequate decompression, recurrent disc herniation, epidural fibrosis (scar tissue formation), incorrect surgical level selection, and spinal instability (Thapa et al., 2023). In some cases, FBSS results from neuropathic pain caused by nerve root damage during surgery, leading to altered pain processing and central sensitization (Kumar et al., 2007).

## Prevalence and Statistics

The prevalence of FBSS varies widely depending on the type of spinal surgery performed, patient selection criteria, and the presence of preexisting conditions.

A meta-analysis reviewing multiple studies estimated that the overall prevalence of FBSS in patients who underwent spinal surgery ranges between 10% and 40%, with higher rates observed in individuals with complex spine conditions such as multi-level degenerative disc disease, failed fusion procedures, or preexisting psychological distress (Manchikanti et al., 2011). These findings suggest that the burden of FBSS extends beyond physical pain, often affecting patients' mental health, quality of life, and economic productivity. A study reported an FBSS incidence rate of 16.8% among 56 patients who underwent open lumbar microdiscectomy (Garg et al., 2022). According to various sources, FBSS affects approximately 10% to 44% of patients who have undergone spinal surgeries, with the incidence varying based on the specific surgical procedure and patient population.

The likelihood of developing FBSS also increases with repeated spinal surgeries. Research indicates that while over 50% of patients experience relief after their first spinal surgery, the success rate declines significantly with subsequent procedures: 30% after the second, 15% after the third, and merely 5% after the fourth surgery (Schultz et al., 2021). This trend highlights the diminishing returns of surgical intervention for chronic back pain and underscores the importance of careful patient selection and conservative treatment options before considering additional surgeries.FBSS remains a significant challenge in spine surgery, with varying rates of occurrence depending on surgical techniques, patient selection, and preexisting conditions.

**Conclusion**

While different types of back pain originate from varying structural issues, the key to proper treatment is understanding where the body is stuck in the healing cycle. Rather than focusing solely on the diagnosis or the location of pain, effective recovery depends on facilitating the body's transition through inflammation, proliferation, and maturation. Addressing inflammation, supporting tissue healing, and promoting long-term structural adaptation are the most important aspects of restoring function and achieving lasting relief.

Navigating The Healing Journey: How Your Body Recovers Naturally

## The Body's Healing Process and Chronic Back Pain

Understanding the normal body healing process is essential for effectively treating chronic back pain, as persistent pain is often linked to systemic imbalances, inflammation, and impaired recovery mechanisms. The body's natural healing cycle involves recognition, response, repair, and restoration. When an injury or musculoskeletal imbalance occurs, the body initiates an inflammatory response to address the issue, followed by cellular repair and tissue regeneration. However, chronic back pain may result from dysregulated healing processes, where persistent inflammation, nervous system hypersensitivity, and structural dysfunction interfere with the body's ability to restore balance. These disruptions prevent normal recovery, leading to recurring pain episodes and prolonged discomfort.

Research suggests that individuals with chronic back pain often exhibit impaired mitochondrial function, oxidative stress, and neurovascular dysregulation, which can hinder normal healing mechanisms. These disruptions contribute to prolonged pain cycles and increased sensitivity to movement and pressure. Understanding how the body heals and identifying factors that interfere with this process, such as nutrient deficiencies, chronic stress, and fascial restrictions, are essential for effective treatment. By implementing targeted strategies, recovery can be enhanced, inflammation reduced, and musculoskeletal balance restored.

The normal healing cycle consists of three stages, which can be illustrated using an external paper cut to visualize what happens internally in the body. See the image above for more details. The first stage is inflammation, characterized by swelling, redness, pain, and increased blood flow to the affected area. The second stage involves the formation of fibrosis, also known as scar tissue, which fills the wound to prevent it from remaining open and susceptible to infection. During this stage, the injured site may also experience fascial restrictions and muscle spasms. This highlights the essential role of scar tissue in our protection and survival.

The third stage of the healing cycle involves the breakdown of fibrotic tissue. Ideally, in a perfect world with perfect bodies, the body would autonomously break down this fibrotic tissue over a period of days, weeks, or months, depending on the severity of the injury. However, we do not live in a perfect

## Normal Healing Cycle

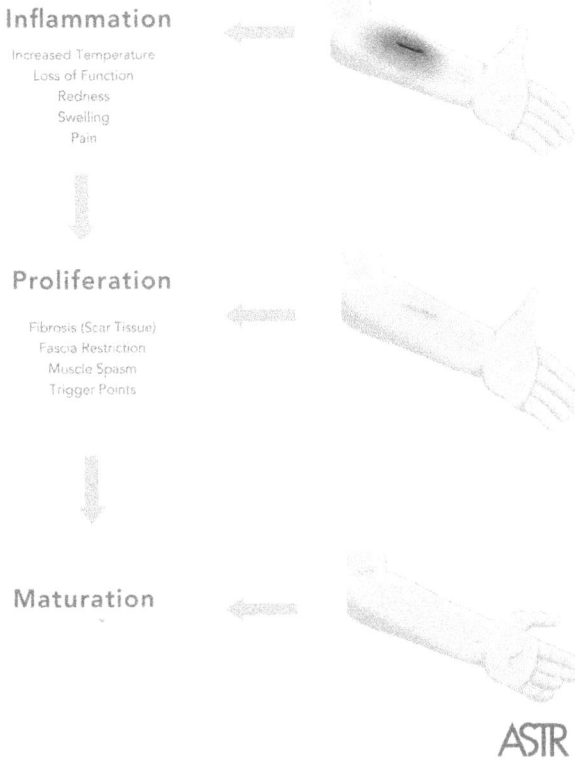

### Inflammation

Increased Temperature
Loss of Function
Redness
Swelling
Pain

### Proliferation

Fibrosis (Scar Tissue)
Fascia Restriction
Muscle Spasm
Trigger Points

### Maturation

ASTR

world. As we age, our body's ability to break down scar tissue decreases significantly.

This healing process also occurs internally when our bodies experience injuries from accidents, surgeries, trauma, poor posture, or stress. Below, the normal muscle healing process after injury is described in more depth, outlining a complex sequence that can be divided into several overlapping phases. The duration of each phase can vary depending on the severity of the injury and the individual's overall health. In chronic conditions, the injured area may not progress through all three stages, instead getting stuck between the inflammation and proliferation stages. Here is a breakdown of the normal muscle healing cycle:

**Destruction Stage (Injury Initiation)**

This initial phase begins immediately after injury and is characterized by the disruption of muscle fibers and blood vessels, leading to the formation of a hematoma (a localized collection of blood outside of blood vessels). The hematoma serves to contain the damage and forms a scaffold for incoming inflammatory cells.

## 1. Inflammatory Stage
This phase starts within hours after the injury and can last for several days. It involves the following key processes:

- **Inflammation**: In response to injury, inflammatory cells such as neutrophils and macrophages infiltrate the site. They remove debris, damaged cells, and pathogens. This phase is associated with the classic signs of inflammation: redness, heat, swelling, and pain.
- **Release of Cytokines**: Inflammatory cells release cytokines and growth factors that are crucial for healing and recruiting more reparative cells to the injury site.

## 2. Proliferation Stage
During this phase, the focus shifts from clearing out the debris to rebuilding muscle tissue, and typically lasts from several days to a couple of weeks:

- **Myogenesis**: This is the formation of new muscle fibers through the activation, differentiation, and fusion of myoblasts (muscle progenitor cells).
- **Fibroblast Proliferation**: Fibroblasts produce collagen and other extracellular matrix components that form the scar tissue, providing structural integrity to the healing muscle. During this stage, fibrosis (scar tissue) closes the injured site and adheres the fascial layers together, causing fascial restrictions. I will discuss fascial restrictions in depth in the chapter on fascial restriction.
- **Angiogenesis**: New blood vessels form to provide necessary nutrients and oxygen to the regenerating tissue.

## 3. Maturation Stage: The Remodeling Phase

This final phase can last from several weeks to months and is focused on strengthening and refining the newly formed tissue:

- **Maturation of Muscle Fibers**: Newly formed muscle fibers mature and increase in size and strength.
- **Collagen Remodeling**: The initially disorganized collagen fibers become more organized and aligned along the lines of stress, which improves the tensile strength of the muscle.
- **Functional Recovery**: Gradually, the muscle regains its strength and functionality, although the healed muscle may never completely return to its pre-injury state.

## Factors Influencing Muscle Healing

Several factors can affect the efficiency and outcome of muscle healing, including:

- **Age**: Younger individuals tend to heal faster than older adults.
- **Malnutrition**
- **Vitamins, Minerals, and Hormonal Imbalances**
- **Blood Supply**: Muscles with good blood supply generally heal better than those with less vascularization.
- **Re-injury**: Avoiding re-injury during the healing process is crucial for successful recovery.
- **Poor Posture and Body Mechanics**

## Chronic Condition Vicious Cycle

According to the U.S. National Center for Health Statistics, a chronic condition is typically defined as one that persists for three months or more. In a chronic condition, the injured body part becomes trapped in a vicious cycle, continuously oscillating between the inflammation and proliferation stages. This cycle leads to excessive inflammation and fibrosis, which in turn cause muscle spasms and severe fascial restrictions. Deficiencies in vitamins and minerals can cause the body to remain stuck in the inflammation-proliferation cycle,

# Chronic Conditions

## Inflammation

Increased Temperature
Loss of Function
Redness
Swelling
Pain

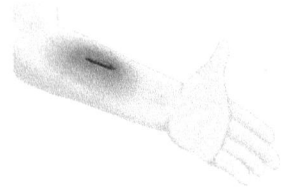

## Proliferation

Fibrosis (Scar Tissue)
Fascia Restriction
Muscle Spasm
Trigger Points

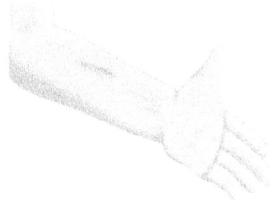

ASTR

preventing progression to the maturation stage. Additionally, excessive fibrosis and severe fascial restrictions can further complicate the issue, making it harder to break the cycle of chronic back pain.

When essential nutrients are lacking, the body's ability to regulate inflammation, repair tissues, and restore normal function is compromised. Deficiencies in key vitamins and minerals disrupt cellular energy production, weaken the immune system, and impair the body's ability to detoxify, further fueling chronic inflammation.

Chronic stress further exacerbates this cycle by increasing cortisol levels, which can dysregulate the immune system, disrupt hormone balance, and intensify inflammation. Elevated stress hormones place the nervous system in a constant state of overactivity, making the body more susceptible to pain and reducing its ability to recover from back pain episodes. Additionally, poor posture and musculoskeletal imbalances contribute to fascial restrictions and tension, further stimulating pain pathways and delaying the body's transition to the maturation stage of healing.

The maturation stage is the final phase of tissue repair, where collagen is properly remodeled, inflammation subsides, and the body fully recovers. However, without sufficient vitamins, minerals, and targeted interventions, the body remains stuck in a state of chronic dysfunction, unable to complete the healing cycle. Instead of progressing to full recovery, the body continuously cycles through inflammation and proliferation, leading to persistent pain, tissue dysfunction, and ongoing back pain episodes.

In order to break this vicious cycle and effectively treat back pain, it is essential to address the seven elements presented in this book, which are designed to restore balance, reduce inflammation, and promote long-term healing. By optimizing nutrition, correcting postural imbalances, managing stress, and supporting the body's natural healing mechanisms, individuals can transition from chronic pain and inflammation to full recovery and musculoskeletal stability. Properly nourishing the body with the right balance of vitamins and minerals is a crucial step in allowing it to move beyond the inflammatory phase and complete the healing process.

# 1. Inflammatory Foods

Chronic back pain is a prevalent condition that can be influenced by various factors, including dietary habits. Emerging research indicates that certain foods may exacerbate inflammation, potentially contributing to or worsening back pain. Understanding the relationship between diet and inflammation is crucial for developing effective strategies to manage and alleviate back pain.

**Pro-Inflammatory Foods and Their Impact on Back Pain**

Several dietary components have been identified as pro-inflammatory, potentially aggravating back pain:

## 1. Sugar and High-Fructose Corn Syrup

High intakes of sugar and high-fructose corn syrup can exacerbate inflammation, oxidative stress, and insulin resistance. These sweeteners are prevalent in many processed foods and beverages. Sugar consumption can increase inflammation and contribute to insulin resistance, thereby intensifying pain and swelling in joints. Common sources include soft drinks, candies, and various desserts.

Research by Sanchez et al. on the impact of carbohydrates, including glucose, on the phagocytic capacity of neutrophils in normal human subjects revealed that simple carbohydrates significantly decrease the capacity of neutrophils to engulf bacteria, with effects lasting for at least five hours post-ingestion.

Engulfing bacteria is a process known as phagocytosis, where certain cells of the immune system, primarily phagocytes such as neutrophils and macrophages, ingest and destroy bacteria and other foreign particles. This suggests that **glucose can induce internal inflammation lasting for five hours**. Consuming three meals a day that contain refined carbs or simple sugars could subject the body to 15 hours of internal inflammation daily. Over a year, this means the body could be in a state of inflammation most of the time.

## 2. Artificial Trans Fats

These are considered the most unhealthy fats, created by adding hydrogen to unsaturated fats, which are found in margarine, spreads, and various processed foods. Trans fats are linked to increased inflammation, heart disease, and other health problems. Foods containing trans fats, especially artificial trans fats like margarine, are known to promote inflammation. These fats are often present in processed snacks and baked goods (Shin et al., 2022).

## 3. Vegetable and Seed Oils

Some vegetable oils that are high in omega-6 fatty acids and low in omega-3 fatty acids can contribute to inflammation if consumed in large quantities. Examples include corn, safflower, sunflower, and soybean oils. These oils tend to promote inflammation when consumed in large amounts, especially if the balance between omega-6 and omega-3 fatty acids in the diet is skewed towards omega-6s. Consumption of omega-6 fatty acids, commonly found in vegetable oils such as corn, safflower, soybean, and sunflower oils, can promote inflammatory processes (Shin et al., 2022).

## 4. Refined Carbohydrates

Foods made from refined grains are stripped of their fiber and most nutrients during processing. When consumed, they can lead to rapid spikes in blood sugar and insulin levels. These spikes can, in turn, trigger an inflammatory response. Chronic high blood sugar levels can lead to insulin resistance, which is linked to further inflammation. Over time, this ongoing low-grade inflammation can contribute to the development of chronic diseases such as type 2 diabetes, heart disease, and other inflammatory conditions.

High intake of refined and simple carbohydrates has been associated with an increased risk of metabolic diseases and negative effects on mental health, including mood disorders like anxiety and depression. Reducing the intake of refined carbohydrates and replacing them with whole grain options can help manage and reduce inflammation. High consumption of sugars and refined carbohydrates, such as those found in pastries, white bread, and sugary beverages, can lead to increased inflammation. These foods cause rapid spikes in blood sugar levels, triggering inflammatory responses (Shin et al., 2022).

## 5. Processed Foods

Diets high in processed foods have been linked to increased inflammation, potentially exacerbating back pain. A cross-sectional study involving 7,686 Kurdish adults identified an "energy-dense" dietary pattern—characterized by high consumption of sweets, desserts, hydrogenated fats, soft drinks, refined grains, tea, and coffee—which was associated with higher odds of chronic low back pain (OR: 1.13, 95% CI: 1.01–1.32) (Mansouri et al., 2022).

## 6. Dairy Products

For individuals with lactose intolerance or dairy sensitivities, consumption of dairy products can trigger inflammation, leading to digestive issues and systemic inflammation. This inflammatory response may contribute to musculoskeletal discomfort, including back pain (Mahan & Escott-Stump, 2008).

## 7. Alcohol

Excessive alcohol intake has been associated with increased inflammatory responses, negatively impacting overall health and potentially worsening back pain. Alcohol consumption can lead to gut inflammation and has been linked to conditions such as pancreatitis, which manifests as abdominal and back pain (Yadav & Lowenfels, 2013).

## 8. Caffeine

While moderate caffeine consumption is generally considered safe, excessive intake may elevate stress hormones like cortisol, potentially increasing inflammation and exacerbating back pain. High caffeine consumption has been associated with increased risk of musculoskeletal disorders (Shiri et al., 2013).

## Recommendations for Dietary Modifications

To mitigate inflammation and potentially reduce back pain, individuals are advised to:

- **Limit Intake of Pro-Inflammatory Foods**: Reducing consumption of sugars, refined carbohydrates, trans fats, excessive omega-6 fatty acids, processed foods, dairy products (if lactose intolerant), excessive alcohol, and caffeine can help decrease inflammation.

- **Adopt an Anti-Inflammatory Diet**: Emphasizing a diet rich in fruits, vegetables, whole grains, proteins, and healthy fats (such as omega-3 fatty acids found in fish) can help reduce inflammation.

- **Stay Hydrated**: Adequate water intake is essential for overall health and can help reduce inflammation.

## ASTR Diet:

Following an anti-inflammatory diet is crucial for managing back pain, as it helps reduce internal inflammation and supports the body's natural healing process. Chronic inflammation can keep the body stuck in the early stages of healing, preventing proper tissue repair and leading to persistent pain. Many processed foods, refined sugars, and unhealthy fats contribute to systemic inflammation, making it harder for the body to recover. By adopting an anti-inflammatory approach, individuals can create an environment that promotes tissue regeneration, reduces pain, and enhances overall well-being.

One of the most effective ways to implement an anti-inflammatory diet is by following the ASTR Diet, which stands for Anti-inflammatory, Sustainable, Toxin-free, and Restorative. Each component plays a critical role in supporting the body's ability to heal. The Anti-inflammatory aspect focuses on incorporating whole foods such as leafy greens, healthy fats, and antioxidant-rich fruits, which help lower systemic inflammation. The Sustainable element ensures that dietary choices promote long-term health while considering environmental impact, emphasizing organic and minimally processed foods. The Toxin-free principle eliminates harmful additives, pesticides, and chemicals that can contribute to chronic inflammation and interfere with the body's healing process. Lastly, the Restorative aspect prioritizes nutrient-dense foods, balanced macronutrient intake, and intermittent fasting to support cellular repair and optimize metabolic function.

# 1.Inflammatory Foods

Since nutrition plays a foundational role in reducing back pain and optimizing musculoskeletal health, it is difficult to cover all aspects of the ASTR Diet in just one chapter. A complete guide on how to implement this diet effectively, including detailed meal plans and strategies for long-term health, can be found in **Eat to Heal.** This book provides a deeper understanding of how dietary changes can accelerate healing, reduce inflammation, and improve overall physical function. For those looking to take a proactive approach to back pain relief, adopting the principles of the ASTR Diet can be a powerful step toward lasting recovery.

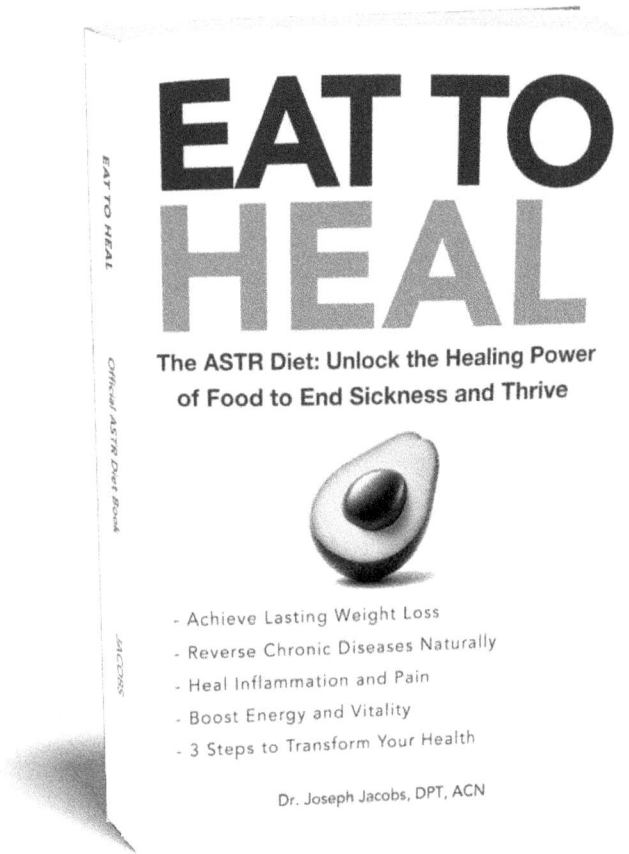

# EAT TO HEAL

**The ASTR Diet: Unlock the Healing Power of Food to End Sickness and Thrive**

- Achieve Lasting Weight Loss
- Reverse Chronic Diseases Naturally
- Heal Inflammation and Pain
- Boost Energy and Vitality
- 3 Steps to Transform Your Health

Dr. Joseph Jacobs, DPT, ACN

EAT TO HEAL

Official ASTR Diet Book

JACOBS

## 2. Vitamin, Mineral, and Hormonal Imbalances

Back pain is a complex musculoskeletal condition influenced by various factors, including deficiencies in specific vitamins, minerals, and hormones. Research has identified several nutrient deficiencies that may contribute to the onset and severity of chronic back pain. However, because each individual's biochemistry is unique, it is essential to work with a clinical nutritionist to conduct comprehensive lab testing to identify specific deficiencies and determine the appropriate dosage of supplementation. Treating back pain effectively requires a customized approach, as lab values and nutritional needs differ from person to person.

## Vitamin D Deficiency

Vitamin D plays a critical role in modulating inflammation and maintaining musculoskeletal health. A deficiency in vitamin D has been associated with an increased risk of chronic back pain. A study by Glover et al. (2021) found that individuals with lower serum levels of vitamin D experienced higher pain intensity and reduced mobility, suggesting that inadequate vitamin D levels contribute to prolonged and severe back pain. Further research indicates that vitamin D influences bone density, muscle function, and inflammatory pathways, which are often dysregulated in individuals suffering from chronic back pain. Proper supplementation, based on individual lab results, may help reduce pain frequency and intensity (Glover et al., 2021). Optimal dosing requires lab-guided monitoring, as excessive vitamin D may lead to hypercalcemia, kidney strain, and increased cardiovascular risk.

## Magnesium Deficiency

Magnesium is essential for numerous physiological processes, including muscle function, nerve conduction, and neurotransmitter regulation. Low magnesium levels have been linked to increased muscle tension, spasms, and chronic pain syndromes, including lower back pain. Research indicates that magnesium deficiency is common among individuals with chronic back pain, and lower serum magnesium levels are correlated with increased pain severity (Jahromi et al., 2019). A double-blind study found that magnesium supplementation significantly reduced muscle tightness and back pain intensity by up to 40%, further confirming its role in musculoskeletal health (Peikert et al., 1996). However, excessive magnesium intake can cause gastrointestinal distress, making personalized dosing through lab testing essential. Optimal dosing should be based on individual laboratory findings to ensure effective levels without unnecessary side effects. Excessive intake may cause gastrointestinal symptoms, confusion, cardiac arrest, and kidney dysfunction, emphasizing the need for personalized dosing.

## Riboflavin (Vitamin B2) Deficiency

Riboflavin is crucial for mitochondrial energy production, and mitochondrial dysfunction has been proposed as a contributing factor in chronic pain conditions. A systematic review of randomized controlled trials concluded that riboflavin supplementation significantly reduced muscle fatigue and pain intensity in individuals with chronic musculoskeletal pain (Thompson et al., 2017). Because riboflavin is water-soluble, excess amounts are excreted in urine, making it a generally safe option. However, optimal dosing should be based on individual laboratory findings to ensure effective levels without unnecessary supplementation.

## Cobalamin (Vitamin B12) Deficiency

Vitamin B12, also known as cobalamin, is essential for nerve function and red blood cell formation. Emerging research suggests a potential link between vitamin B12 deficiency and chronic back pain. A study by Üstün Özek (2022) found that patients with chronic back pain had significantly lower vitamin B12 levels compared to those with less frequent pain episodes. This negative correlation indicates that vitamin B12 deficiency may contribute to increased pain sensitivity and nerve dysfunction. Similarly, a case-control study by Ghorbani et al. (2019) reported that chronic pain patients exhibited significantly lower serum vitamin B12 levels, suggesting that lower functional activity of vitamin B12 is associated with a higher likelihood of experiencing chronic back pain. Regular monitoring and appropriate supplementation of vitamin B12 may serve as a beneficial component in the holistic management of back pain. Excessive intake may cause numbness, burning sensations, and itching, emphasizing the need for personalized dosing.

## Iron Deficiency

Iron is essential for oxygen transport and energy production. A study by Özdemir et al. (2018) found that low ferritin levels were significantly associated with an increased risk of chronic back pain, particularly in menstruating women. Iron deficiency anemia can lead to hypoxia (low oxygen levels), which may contribute to muscular pain and fatigue. However, excess iron can be harmful, leading to oxidative stress and organ damage. Proper lab testing is crucial to assess iron levels before supplementation.

## Zinc Deficiency

Zinc is a critical mineral involved in immune function, neurotransmitter activity, and inflammation regulation. Recent studies suggest that low zinc levels may contribute to chronic pain susceptibility by affecting neuroinflammatory pathways (Yabanlı & Özer, 2022). Zinc supplementation has shown promise in pain management, but excess intake can interfere with copper absorption, highlighting the importance of individualized lab assessments.

## Estrogen and Progesterone Imbalances

Hormonal fluctuations, particularly in estrogen and progesterone levels, can contribute to chronic back pain, especially in women. Estrogen influences bone density, muscle function, and neurotransmitter activity, which are all implicated in pain perception. Research by Martin & Behbehani (2006) found that estrogen withdrawal (as seen in menopause) can lead to increased pain sensitivity and musculoskeletal discomfort. Additionally, low progesterone levels relative to estrogen (estrogen dominance) may further contribute to back pain. Hormone testing can help determine whether dietary modifications or lifestyle interventions are necessary for balancing hormones and reducing chronic pain.

## Thyroid Hormone Imbalances

Hypothyroidism (low thyroid hormone levels) has been associated with an increased risk of chronic musculoskeletal pain, including back pain. A study by Gökmen-Yıldırım et al. (2020) found that individuals with hypothyroidism had a significantly higher prevalence of chronic pain compared to those with normal thyroid function. The exact mechanism remains unclear, but thyroid dysfunction may contribute to pain through metabolic dysregulation and impaired neurotransmitter function. Proper thyroid function testing, including TSH, free T3, and free T4, is essential for determining whether thyroid imbalances contribute to chronic pain.

## Conclusion

Based on my clinical experience, I have observed that patients experiencing **back pain commonly suffer from deficiencies in approximately three to six essential vitamins and minerals.** These deficiencies frequently involve key nutrients such as vitamin D, magnesium, zinc, and B vitamins, all of which play crucial roles in musculoskeletal health. Deficiencies in these nutrients can exacerbate inflammation, compromise muscle function, and impair bone density, ultimately contributing to chronic back pain and delayed recovery. It is important to collaborate with a clinical nutritionist to accurately assess your vitamin and mineral levels and to establish customized supplementation dosages. Addressing these nutritional gaps through targeted dietary adjustments and supplementation has often proven beneficial, resulting in significant pain relief and improved patient outcomes.

Addressing deficiencies in vitamins, minerals, and hormones through comprehensive lab testing and individualized supplementation is a powerful strategy for managing chronic back pain naturally. While generalized supplementation may help some individuals, a personalized approach based on lab values ensures that the right nutrients are provided at the correct dosages. By identifying and correcting nutrient and hormonal imbalances, individuals can take a proactive approach to reducing pain severity and improving overall well-being.

## 3. Posture

## The Role of Poor Posture in Back Pain

Poor posture, particularly involving the neck and spine, has been implicated in the development and exacerbation of chronic back pain. Forward head posture (FHP), characterized by the anterior positioning of the head relative to the spine, is a common postural deviation that increases muscle tension in the neck, shoulders, and lower back, potentially triggering chronic pain episodes. A study by Yip et al. (2008) found that individuals with chronic neck and back pain exhibited a higher prevalence of FHP compared to asymptomatic controls, suggesting a link between this postural misalignment and musculoskeletal disorders.

Further research indicates that back pain is highly prevalent among individuals with poor posture. A cross-sectional study by Jun et al. (2017) reported that 68.9% of participants with chronic back pain demonstrated significant postural misalignments, including excessive lumbar lordosis and forward head positioning. The study concluded that improper posture is significantly associated with increased back pain intensity, highlighting the importance of addressing spinal musculoskeletal factors in pain management.

From my personal experience treating patients with chronic back pain, I have consistently observed that they also suffer from tension and muscle strain, which are often caused and triggered by poor posture, fibrotic tissue, and fascial restrictions. Poor neck and spinal posture, particularly forward head posture and slouched sitting, can increase stress on the vertebrae and intervertebral discs. This increased stress may lead to compression of the spinal nerves, reducing mobility and exacerbating pain. Many of my patients have reported significant improvement in their back pain symptoms after addressing these postural issues through manual therapy, postural correction exercises, and fascial release techniques. Below are detailed tips on how to maintain proper posture and body mechanics.

## Posture and Body Mechanics Training Videos Available Online.

**Standing Posture**
1.   **Visualize a string**: Imagine a string coming out of the top of your head, pulling you upward towards the ceiling.
2.   **Core engagement**: Keep your belly button sucked in.

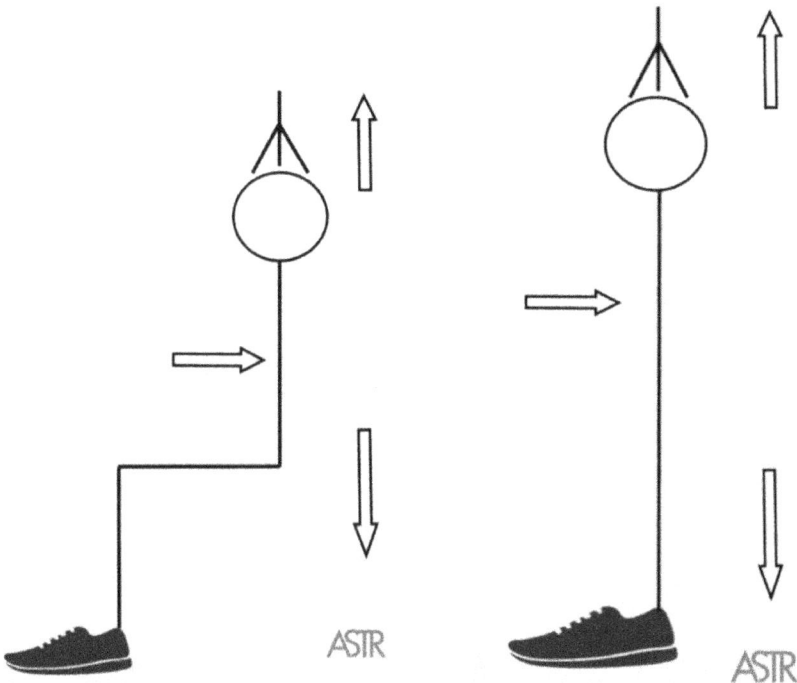

3.   **Feet positioning**: Feet should be shoulder-width apart, with weight distributed through your heels.

**Sitting Posture**
1.   **Visualize a string**: Imagine a string coming out of the top of your head, pulling you upward towards the ceiling.
2.   **Engage your core**: Keep your belly button sucked in.
3.   **Proper weight distribution**: Distribute your weight through your buttocks; keep your feet flat and shoulder-width apart.

**Walking Posture**

Posture

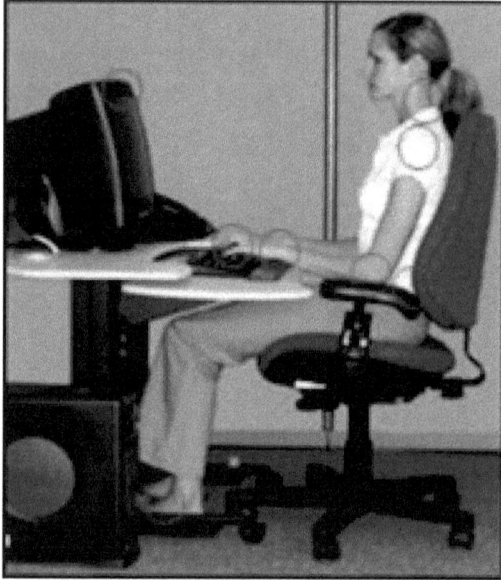

1. **Visualize a string**: Imagine a string coming out of the top of your head, pulling you upward towards the ceiling.
2. **Engage your core**: Suck your belly button in to stabilize your spine.

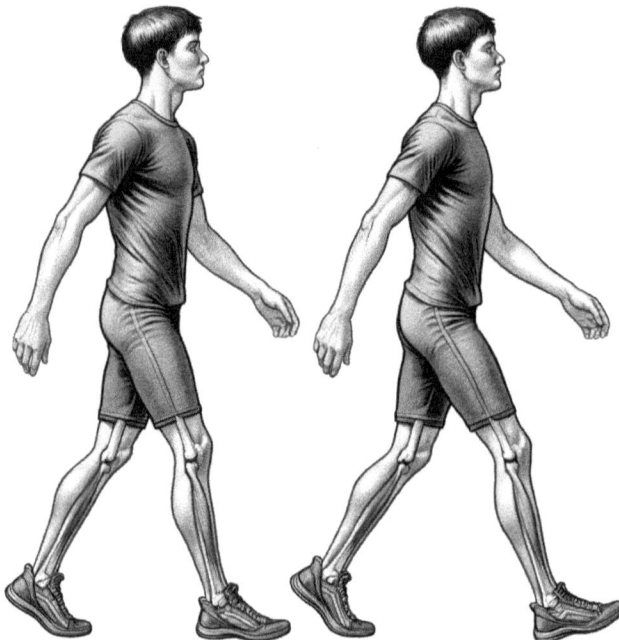

3.  **Heel first**: Ensure your heel touches the ground first, then roll through to your toes.

**General Tips**
- **Start gradually**: Begin with short intervals, and progressively increase the duration you maintain these postures.
- **Be mindful**: Regularly check in with your body to ensure you're maintaining proper posture.
- **Create reminders**: Setting reminders can help you remember to adjust your posture throughout the day.

**Correct Computer Posture**
1.  **Head and Neck Alignment**: Imagine a string pulling upward from the top of your head, keeping it level or slightly forward-facing and aligned with your torso. The neck should remain neutral, avoiding any tilting or twisting.
2.  **Shoulder and Arm Position**: Shoulders should be relaxed, with upper arms hanging naturally at your sides. Elbows should be close to the body and bent at a 90-degree angle. Hands, wrists, and forearms should be straight, in-line, and roughly parallel to the floor, with forearms comfortably supported by armrests.
3.  **Back Support**: Ensure your back is fully supported by the chair. Whether sitting upright or leaning back slightly, avoid twisting the back.
4.  **Seat Positioning**: Thighs and hips should be supported by a well-padded seat, generally parallel to the floor. Knees should be at about the same height as the hips, with feet slightly forward.
5.  **Foot Support**: Feet should rest fully on the floor. If the desk height is not adjustable and your feet do not comfortably reach the floor, use a footrest or a book to provide support.
6.  **Monitor Setup**: Place the computer monitor directly in front of you, at eye level, to avoid straining your neck. The screen should be about an arm's length away, ensuring you do not have to tilt your head up, down, or sideways.

**Additional Tips:**
- **Adjust your chair**: Make sure your chair height and backrest are adjustable to fit your body dimensions.

- **Take breaks**: Regularly stand up, stretch, and walk around to relieve muscle tension and improve circulation.
- **Monitor brightness and distance**: Adjust the brightness of your monitor to a comfortable level to reduce eye strain. Ensure the monitor is neither too close nor too far for comfortable viewing.
- **Workspace layout**: Keep frequently used objects within easy reach to minimize reaching and twisting.

Implementing these practices can help reduce the risk of strain and discomfort. This contributes to a healthier, more productive work environment.

## TV/Reading Posture

1. **Head and Neck Alignment**: Keep your head level or bent slightly forward, ensuring it remains in line with your torso. Your neck should be in a neutral position, not tilted to the side or excessively up or down.
2. **Eye Level**: Position your book or TV screen straight in front of you at eye level. This setup helps prevent neck strain by eliminating the need to look too far up, down, or to the side.
3. **Use a Reading Stand**: For reading, use a stand to hold your book. This reduces the strain on your arms and helps maintain a better neck posture.
4. **Shoulder Positioning**: Shoulders should be relaxed with upper arms hanging naturally at the sides. Avoid hunching or elevating your shoulders, which can lead to tension.
5. **Back Support**: Ensure your back is fully supported by the chair or sofa. Whether sitting upright or leaning back slightly, avoid twisting the back. This supports the natural curve of your spine and reduces lower back strain.
6. **Arm and Hand Relaxation**:Use a reading stand or rest your forearm on a pillow so that your hands and arms can rest comfortably. This reduces the strain of holding up a book for long periods.

## Additional Recommendations:

- **Lighting**: Ensure adequate lighting for reading to avoid eye strain. The light source should come from behind you, ideally over your shoulder, to illuminate the page or screen without causing glare.

- **Seating Choice**: Choose a comfortable chair or sofa that supports your posture with cushions if necessary. Consider a recliner or a chair with an adjustable back for added comfort.
- **Take Breaks**: Regularly change your position and take breaks to stretch and move around. This helps reduce muscle fatigue and stiffness from prolonged sitting.

Implementing these recommendations can greatly enhance your viewing and reading experience, promoting better posture and reducing the risk of discomfort or injury.

### Correct Back Sleeping Posture

1. **Avoid Stomach Sleeping**: Sleeping on your stomach can put excessive strain on your neck and back. Instead, opt for back sleeping as it supports natural spinal alignment.
2. **Head and Neck Alignment**: Keep your head in a neutral position,

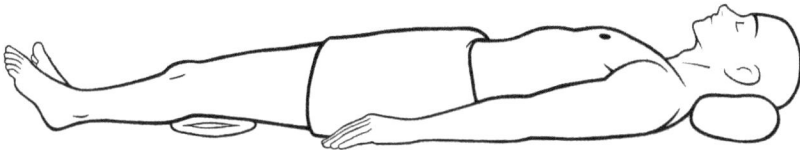

avoiding any flexion (tilting forward) or excessive side bending. Use a semi-firm contoured memory foam pillow that supports the natural curve of your neck.
3. **Knee Support**: To maintain better spinal alignment and relieve pressure on your lower back, place a pillow under your knees. This helps flatten the lumbar region against the mattress and reduces stress on the spine.

### Additional Tips:

- **Mattress Selection**: Choose a mattress that supports the contour of your spine. It should be firm enough to support your body but soft enough to allow for slight sinking of the heavier parts of your body.
- **Pillow Adjustments**: Ensure your pillow is not too high. It should just fill the space between your neck and the mattress to maintain proper alignment without lifting your head too high.

- **Relaxation Before Bed**: Engaging in relaxation techniques such as deep breathing before bed can help reduce muscle tension and promote better sleep.
- **Regular Review**: Evaluate your sleeping environment regularly to ensure it continues to meet your needs. This is especially important if you experience changes in health or comfort.

Implementing these practices not only improves your posture during sleep but can also enhance sleep quality. This helps prevent common discomforts associated with poor sleeping positions.

### Correct Side Sleeping Posture

1. **Avoid Stomach Sleeping**: Sleeping on your stomach is discouraged due to potential neck and back strain. Side sleeping is a healthier alternative that supports better spinal alignment.
2. **Head and Neck Support**: Keep your head in a neutral position, avoiding any forward flexion or side bending. Use a semi-firm contoured memory foam pillow that adequately supports the natural curve of your neck. This aligns it with the rest of your spine.

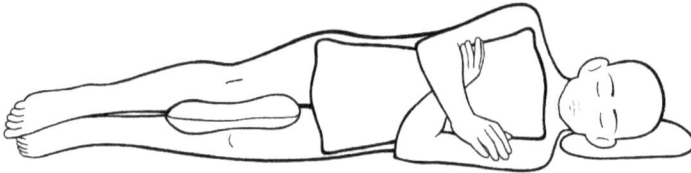

3. **Knee and Hip Alignment**: Place a pillow thick enough between your knees to ensure that your hips, knees, and ankles are aligned. This prevents the upper leg from pulling the spine out of alignment and reduces stress on the hips and lower back.
4. **Avoid Trunk Twisting**: Maintain your trunk in a straight alignment with your hips and shoulders stacked directly above each other. This prevents any twisting. Ensure your hips, knees, and ankles remain directly on top of each other.
5. **Use a Body Pillow**: A body pillow can be beneficial for side sleepers. It provides support for the arms and the entire body, helping to stabilize the trunk and prevent it from twisting during the night.

**Additional Tips:**

- **Pillow Adjustments**: Adjust the height and firmness of your pillow to ensure it fills the gap between your shoulder and the mattress. This helps maintain a straight neck and spine.
- **Mattress Firmness**: Choose a mattress that supports your body's weight while cushioning pressure points like hips and shoulders.
- **Regular Position Changes**: If feasible, alternate sides throughout the night to avoid overuse and strain on one side of your body.
- **Relaxation Techniques**: Engage in relaxing activities such as reading before bed to prepare your body for restful sleep.

Implementing these posture guidelines can greatly improve your sleep quality and contribute to overall spinal health.

# 4. Stress Management

**The Link Between Stress and Back Pain**

Stress is one of the most commonly reported contributors to chronic back pain, with research indicating that psychological stress can exacerbate pain perception and muscular tension (American Psychological Association, 2021). Studies have shown that individuals experiencing high levels of stress are more likely to develop back pain, and stress-related muscle tension can contribute to prolonged discomfort and reduced mobility (van der Meulen et al., 2020).

Fluctuations in stress levels, rather than stress itself, may play a significant role in pain intensity. A study published in Pain Medicine found that individuals who experienced stress fluctuations had a greater likelihood of developing back pain episodes due to increased muscle activation and tension (Davis et al., 2018). This suggests that the body's response to stress, rather than stress itself, plays a crucial role in the development and persistence of back pain.

The physiological mechanisms linking stress and back pain involve activation of the hypothalamic-pituitary-adrenal (HPA) axis, which regulates the body's stress response. During periods of acute stress, the body releases cortisol and other stress-related hormones, which have been found at elevated levels in individuals with chronic pain (Kim, 2024). Dysregulation of the HPA axis can contribute to heightened pain sensitivity and increased neuroinflammation, worsening chronic back pain (Borsook et al., 2012). Chronic stress has also been associated with increased central sensitization, a condition in which the nervous system becomes more sensitive to pain stimuli, leading to prolonged and intensified back pain symptoms (Sauro & Becker, 2009).

Beyond physiological mechanisms, stress may also reduce the effectiveness of back pain treatments. Research indicates that individuals with higher levels of perceived stress often experience poorer responses to physical therapy and other pain management interventions (Borsook et al., 2012). Interestingly, minor daily stressors, rather than major life events, appear to have a more substantial impact on back pain occurrence, emphasizing the importance of managing everyday stress in pain prevention and recovery (Sauro & Becker, 2009). Addressing stress through relaxation techniques, mindfulness, and cognitive behavioral therapy can help individuals manage their pain more effectively and support long-term musculoskeletal health.

Research studies showing that stress has consistently demonstrated its impact on various biological systems, potentially leading to a range of health issues. Here's a summary of how stress affects different parts of the body based on scientific studies:

1. Cardiovascular Effects: Stress may increase heart rate, blood pressure, and oxygen demand on the heart. It can also lead to vasoconstriction, increased blood lipids, and blood clotting issues, contributing to atherosclerosis and increased risk of heart attack and stroke.
2. Metabolic Effects: Stress can cause the liver to produce extra blood sugar (glucose), increasing the risk of developing type 2 diabetes
3. Gastrointestinal Effects: Stress can disrupt normal digestive function, leading to issues like heartburn, acid reflux, diarrhea, constipation, and stomach pain
4. Musculoskeletal Effects: Stress can cause muscles to tense up, leading to headaches, back pain, shoulder pain, and body aches.
5. Reproductive Effects: In men, stress can lower testosterone levels and interfere with sperm production and sexual function. In women, stress can disrupt the menstrual cycle.
6. Immune System Effects: Chronic stress can weaken the immune system, increasing susceptibility to infections.
7. Neurological/Psychological Effects: Stress can contribute to conditions like anxiety, depression, and insomnia. It can also impair cognitive function like memory and concentration.

Stress and muscle tension are closely related, and understanding this relationship can help in managing both effectively. Here's how stress leads to muscle tension and the potential long-term effects if it remains unaddressed:

### Mechanisms of Muscle Tension Due to Stress

1. **Fight-or-Flight Response:** When you experience stress, your body's fight-or-flight response is triggered. This response prepares your body to either fight or flee from perceived threats. As part of this response, your muscles tense up, readying you for physical action. This was useful in ancient times when physical threats were common. However, in

modern life, this response can be triggered by non-physical stresses like deadlines, traffic, or personal conflicts.

2. **Cortisol Release**: Stress stimulates the release of cortisol, a hormone that increases glucose in the bloodstream and enhances the brain's use of glucose. Cortisol also restricts functions that are non-essential in a fight-or-flight situation, such as the immune response. High cortisol levels can lead to sustained muscle tension.

3. **Neuromuscular Reaction**: Stress affects the nervous system, which controls muscle activation. Under stress, the nervous system may keep muscles in a partly contracted state for prolonged periods.

## Effects of Chronic Muscle Tension

1. **Pain and Discomfort**: Prolonged muscle tension can lead to muscle pain and discomfort, which might manifest as back pain, headaches, or neck pain. Tension-type headaches, one of the most common types of headaches, are directly linked to muscle tension in the neck and scalp.

2. **Reduced Mobility**: Over time, chronic muscle tension can reduce joint mobility. This stiffness can affect your posture and the way you move, potentially leading to mechanical imbalances and injury.

3. **Fibrotic tissue & Trigger Points**: Chronic tension can lead to the development of fibrotic tissue and trigger points—small knots that form in muscles and may cause pain in other parts of the body. These are often tender to the touch and can contribute to pain patterns seen in conditions like myofascial pain syndrome.

4. **Fatigue**: Muscles that are constantly under stress consume energy even when you're at rest. This can lead to muscle fatigue, which reduces your energy levels overall and can impact your physical performance.

## Effective Strategies for Managing Stress

Managing stress effectively is crucial for maintaining both physical and mental health. Here are some practical tips for managing stress:

1. **Identify Stressors**: Keep a journal to identify the situations that create the most stress and how you respond to them. Noting patterns can help you find better coping strategies.

2. **Regular Physical Activity**: Exercise can help alleviate stress by producing endorphins (chemicals in the brain that act as natural painkillers) and improving your ability to sleep, which can reduce stress.

3. **Mindfulness and Meditation**: Techniques such as meditation, deep breathing exercises, and mindfulness can help melt away stress. Start with just a few minutes a day and increase the duration as you feel more comfortable.

4. **Time Management**: Improve your time management skills to avoid feeling overwhelmed. Prioritize tasks, set boundaries, and break projects into manageable steps.

5. **Establish Boundaries**: In today's digital world, it's important to know when to turn off electronic devices. Set boundaries for work and social interactions to ensure personal time for relaxation.

6. **Nourish Your Body**: Eat a healthy diet. Well-nourished bodies are better prepared to cope with stress, so be mindful of what you eat.

7. **Sleep Adequately**: Ensure you get enough sleep. Lack of sleep is a significant contributor to stress. Most adults need 7-9 hours per night.

8. **Connect with Others**: Share your stress and concerns with friends or family members. Social connections can help you feel understood and supported.

9. **Practice Relaxation Techniques**: Engage in activities you enjoy, such as reading, yoga, or listening to music. Try relaxation techniques like progressive muscle relaxation or visualization.

10. **Seek Professional Help**: If your stress levels become too overwhelming, consider seeking professional help. Biopsychosocial therapist can help you learn how to manage stress effectively.

By incorporating these stress management tips into your life, you can find ways to reduce your stress levels and improve your overall well-being.

## Meditation

### Focused Breathing (Eyes Open or Closed)

- **Procedure**: Take a slow, deep breath in and out through your nose, filling your lungs with air.

- **Focus**: Concentrate on your breathing. If your mind wanders, gently redirect it to focus on your breathing.
- **Purpose**: This meditation breathing exercise can be used to help you go to sleep.
- **Session Duration**: 1 to 10 minutes, or as needed throughout the day.

## Breathing Exercise I (Eyes Open)

- **Setting**: Can be done anywhere.
- **Procedure**:
    - Take a slow, deep breath through your nose, filling your lungs with air.
    - Hold your breath for 5 to 15 seconds.
    - Exhale slowly through your nose.
    - Repeat this process 20 times per session.
- **Focus**: Concentrate on your breathing and redirect your focus if your mind wanders.
- **Frequency**: Perform 4-5 sessions per day.

## Breathing Exercise II (Eyes Closed)

- **Setting**: Perform this exercise in a quiet room.
- **Position**: Sit in a comfortable chair with back support, rest your arms on a pillow in your lap, and keep your feet flat on the floor (shoulder width apart).
- **Procedure**:
    - Take a slow, deep breath in through your nose.
    - Hold your breath for 5 to 15 seconds.
    - Exhale slowly through your nose.
    - Repeat this process 20 times per session.
- **Focus**: Concentrate on your breathing and redirect your focus if your mind wanders.
- **Frequency**: Perform 4-5 sessions per day.

## Breathing Exercise III (Eyes Closed)

- **Setting**: Perform this exercise in a quiet room.
- **Position**: Sit in a comfortable chair with back support, rest your arms on a pillow in your lap, and keep your feet flat on the floor (shoulder width apart).

- **Procedure**:
    - Take a slow, deep breath in through your nose.
    - Hold your breath for 5 to 15 seconds.
    - Exhale slowly through your mouth while making a vibration sound.
    - Repeat this process 40 times per session.
- **Focus**: Concentrate on your breathing and redirect your focus if your mind wanders.
- **Frequency**: Perform 2-3 sessions per day.

## Conclusion

While stress is a natural response to life's demands, chronic stress can significantly impact physical health, particularly for those suffering from back pain. Prolonged exposure to stress hormones such as cortisol can lead to inflammation, muscle tension, and a weakened immune response, all of which contribute to persistent pain. That is why learning to manage stress effectively is essential for long-term recovery and overall well-being.

However, when stress progresses into chronic anxiety, depression, or post-traumatic stress disorder (PTSD), a deeper level of support and treatment is needed, one that goes beyond the scope of this chapter. For readers who are facing persistent emotional struggles, I strongly recommend reading my companion book *Beating Anxiety and Depression: 14 Natural Secrets to a Happier Life*. This book is a comprehensive, step-by-step guide that addresses the psychological and biological root causes of emotional distress using clinically proven natural strategies.

Although this chapter offers foundational stress relief tools, the topic of mental health is vast and complex. Attempting to fully address anxiety, depression, and PTSD in a single chapter would not do justice to the depth and individualized care these conditions require. If you or someone you care about is dealing with ongoing emotional pain, I invite you to explore *Beating Anxiety and Depression* as your next step toward healing both mind and body.

# BEATING ANXIETY & DEPRESSION

BONUS VIDEOS

## 14 NATURAL SECRETS TO A HAPPIER LIFE

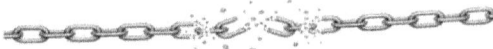

- Conquer Anxiety & Depression Naturally
- Heal the Root Causes & Reclaim Your Life
- Created by a Doctor Who Conquered PTSD & Depression
- Science-Based Strategies for Lasting Change

Dr. Joseph Jacobs, DPT, ACN

BEATING ANXIETY & DEPRESSION

14 NATURAL SECRETS

JACOBS

# 5. Fibrotic Tissue

Do you tend to slouch or hunch forward when using your phone or computer? Believe it or not, poor posture can cause fibrotic tissue (scar tissue) to build up in the neck and shoulders. If possible, place your hand on the back of your shoulder, close to your neck, and press firmly. If you notice a hard knot, it's possible that you have fibrotic tissue (scar tissue) as a result of poor posture. Since we cannot visually see internal fibrotic tissue, it is often overlooked and ignored. Our muscles should act like a rubber band, contracting and relaxing to encourage a full range of motion in the joint. However, fibrotic tissue acts like a knot in the rubber band, limiting its full range of motion. Patients with fibrotic tissue may experience pain and decreased range of motion. If left untreated, this condition can lead to nerve damage, chronic pain, and may even require surgery.

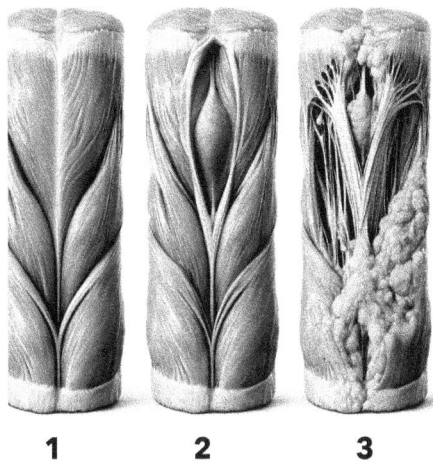

**1**   **2**   **3**

## Image Explanation

1.  **Healthy, intact muscle:** An illustration showing the muscle fibers in their natural, unbroken state.
2.  **Muscle with tear:** An illustration depicting a clear gap in the tissue where the muscle fibers are disrupted and separated.
3.  **Muscle with fibrotic tissue:** An illustration of a muscle with a tear and dense, scar-like fibrotic tissue contrasting with the normal muscle fibers.

## Fibrotic Tissue and Its Role in Back Pain

Back pain is a prevalent musculoskeletal disorder that affects a significant portion of the global population. Recent research suggests that fibrotic tissue changes, characterized by excessive collagen deposition and scarring, contribute to chronic back pain by altering normal tissue function and reducing mobility (Langevin et al., 2011). Fibrosis leads to increased stiffness and decreased elasticity in soft tissues, exacerbating pain and limiting the body's ability to heal properly. This pathological process is particularly evident in cases of post-surgical fibrosis, chronic inflammation, and degenerative spinal conditions.

One key area of concern is the thoracolumbar fascia, a large connective tissue structure in the lower back. Studies indicate that alterations in the mechanical properties of this fascia, particularly increased density and reduced sliding capability, are strongly correlated with chronic low back pain (Wilke et al., 2017). Animal studies have further demonstrated that restricted movement following soft tissue injury can lead to fibrosis and thickening of the thoracolumbar fascia, supporting the hypothesis that fascial adhesions and fibrotic changes contribute to persistent pain (Schilder et al., 2018). This suggests that maintaining fascial mobility through manual therapy, stretching, and movement-based rehabilitation may be crucial in preventing fibrotic tissue from exacerbating back pain.

Post-surgical fibrosis is another major contributor to chronic back pain. Epidural fibrosis, the excessive formation of scar tissue around nerve roots following spinal surgery, is a common factor in failed back surgery syndrome (Bennett et al., 2018). While scar tissue formation is a natural part of the healing process, excessive fibrosis can entrap nerve roots, leading to persistent or recurrent pain. Research indicates that patients who develop epidural fibrosis after laminectomy or discectomy are at significantly higher risk of experiencing long-term pain compared to those with minimal scar tissue formation (Bosscher & Heavner, 2010).

In addition to surgical fibrosis, fibrotic changes have been observed in intervertebral disc degeneration, a primary cause of chronic low back pain. Chronic inflammation is believed to be a key driver of disc fibrosis, as persistent inflammatory signaling leads to excessive extracellular matrix deposition and increased tissue stiffness (Zhao et al., 2021). This process reduces spinal flexibility, alters load distribution, and contributes to mechanical stress, all of which worsen pain over time. Targeting inflammatory pathways through anti-inflammatory diets, physical therapy, and regenerative medicine approaches may offer promising strategies for mitigating fibrosis in degenerative disc disease.

Given the significant role of fibrotic tissue in chronic back pain, addressing fibrosis through targeted interventions is crucial for effective pain management. Therapeutic approaches such as myofascial release, anti-fibrotic medications, platelet-rich plasma (PRP) therapy, and guided movement programs are being explored as potential strategies to reduce fibrotic tissue formation and improve functional outcomes in individuals with chronic back pain (Langevin et al., 2011). Understanding and managing fibrosis at both the physiological and biomechanical levels may provide long-term relief for patients suffering from persistent spinal pain.

## Fibroblasts

Fibroblasts are a type of cell that are essential for wound healing and play a critical role in the maintenance and repair of connective tissues throughout the body. They are the most common cells of connective tissue in animals. They are typically active during the proliferation phase of the healing process. Fibroblasts are a type of cell most commonly found within connective tissues in animals. They play a crucial role in the structural framework of tissues by producing and maintaining the extracellular matrix, which is the complex scaffold of proteins and other substances that support cells. Fibroblasts are responsible for producing key components of this matrix, including collagen, fibronectin, and elastin, which help provide structural integrity and elasticity to tissues.

During wound healing or in response to injury, fibroblasts are activated and multiply. They are crucial in the healing process as they migrate to the site of injury, where they produce collagen and other extracellular matrix components to form fibrotic tissue and repair the damaged tissue. In pathological conditions, fibroblasts can become overly active. This leads to excessive deposition of connective and fibrotic tissue, which can disrupt normal tissue architecture and function.

Here are some key functions and characteristics of fibroblasts:

1. **Tissue Repair and Maintenance**: Fibroblasts produce and secrete collagen and other extracellular matrix proteins that form the structural framework for tissues such as skin, tendons, and ligaments.
2. **Wound Healing**: During the process of wound healing, fibroblasts are activated and migrate to the site of injury. They proliferate and produce collagen and other fibers, which help in closing and healing the wound.
3. **Fibrotic Tissue Formation**: In the proliferation stages of wound healing, fibroblasts help in the formation of fibrotic tissue by depositing excess collagen. This can sometimes lead to the overproduction of fibrosis.
4. **Role in Diseases**: Abnormal function and activation of fibroblasts can contribute to a variety of pathological conditions, including fibrosis (excessive fibrous connective tissue formation) and autoimmune diseases such as rheumatoid arthritis and systemic sclerosis.

Fibroblasts can also differentiate into myofibroblasts, especially during wound healing, which possess contractile capabilities similar to muscle cells, aiding in the contraction of the wound.

### Fibrosis

Fibrosis is defined by the overgrowth, hardening, and/or scarring of various tissues and is attributed to the excess deposition of extracellular matrix components, including collagen. Fibrosis characterizes a pathological state of excessive tissue repair where there is an overgrowth, hardening, and scarring of tissue primarily due to the excessive deposition of extracellular matrix components such as collagen. This process can affect virtually any tissue in the body, leading to significant organ dysfunction depending on the site and severity of the fibrotic response.

Fibrosis often results from chronic inflammatory reactions triggered by a variety of stimuli. These can include:

- **Poor posture and body mechanics:** This is considered a repetitive strain injury due to prolonged poor posture and body mechanics, which cause muscle strain and tendon sprains. This strain leads to inflammation, and eventually, the body builds excessive fibrotic tissue.
- **Persistent infections:** Where ongoing microbial presence provokes a sustained immune response.
- **Autoimmune reactions:** Where the body's immune system mistakenly attacks its own tissues.
- **Allergic responses:** Which can cause chronic inflammation due to repeated exposure to allergens.
- **Chemical insults:** Such as exposure to toxins or irritants that cause tissue damage and subsequent fibrotic repair.
- **Radiation:** Which can damage cells and extracellular matrix, leading to scarring and fibrosis.
- **Physical tissue injury:** From events like trauma or surgery, which initiates the healing process that can sometimes lead to excessive scar tissue formation if the healing process is dysregulated.

The fibrotic process involves complex signaling pathways and cellular interactions, primarily involving fibroblasts, as mentioned earlier. These fibroblasts play a key role in synthesizing and remodeling the extracellular matrix during both normal tissue repair and pathological fibrosis.

Understanding the function of fibroblasts and regulating their activity can be crucial for managing and treating various conditions involving tissue repair and fibrosis. Fibrotic tissue, often known as scar tissue, is a type of connective tissue that forms during the wound healing process, particularly during the proliferation stage. It mainly consists of collagen, a protein that provides structural strength. While essential for repairing damaged areas, excessive fibrotic tissue can lead to muscle or joint pain and restricted range of motion.

### Characteristics of Fibrotic Tissue

1. **Composition**: Fibrotic tissue has a higher density of collagen fibers compared to normal tissue. These fibers are often more disorganized and aligned differently than in the original tissue, which can affect the flexibility and functionality of the area.

2. **Elasticity**: Scar tissue is less elastic and more fibrous than the original tissue. This can lead to stiffness and restricted movement, especially if the fibrosis occurs near joints.
3. **Vascularity**: Fibrotic tissue typically has fewer blood vessels than the original tissue, making it appear paler and potentially leading to a slower metabolic rate in that area.
4. **Sensory Nerves**: fibrotic tissue may have fewer sensory nerves, which can result in areas of numbness or altered sensation.

## Causes of Fibrosis
Fibrosis can result from a variety of conditions and scenarios, including:

- **Injury:** Following trauma or surgery, fibrotic tissue develops as part of the natural healing process to close the wound site. If the wound site remains open, it is susceptible to infection. Fibrotic tissues are crucial for our survival. However, the problem arises when excessive fibrotic tissue forms, which can compress blood vessels and nerves, limit range of motion, and cause pain.
- **Chronic Inflammation**: Diseases that cause long-term inflammation can lead to excessive fibrotic tissue formation. This is seen in conditions such as rheumatoid arthritis, osteoarthritis, fibromyalgia, ankylosing spondylitis, psoriatic arthritis, systemic lupus erythematosus, tendonitis, bursitis, and various autoimmune diseases.
- **Repeated Injury or Irritation**: Areas of the body that undergo repeated stress or injury can become chronically inflamed and subsequently fibrotic.
- **Disease Processes**: Certain diseases can promote fibrosis. These include conditions such as liver cirrhosis from chronic hepatitis or liver damage, pulmonary fibrosis in the lungs, and systemic diseases like scleroderma, which affects connective tissue.
- **Stretching:** Frequent and intense stretching can lead to inflammation and overstimulation of fibroblasts. This can result in increased collagen production and potentially lead to excessive fibrotic tissue formation within the tendons.
- **Poor posture and body mechanics:** This is considered a repetitive strain injury due to prolonged poor posture and body mechanics, which cause muscle strain and tendon sprains. This strain leads to inflammation, and eventually, the body builds excessive fibrotic tissue.

## Impact of Fibrotic Tissue

Excessive fibrotic tissue in the body can have a range of detrimental effects, impacting various organs and systems. Fibrosis is essentially the thickening and scarring of connective tissue, usually resulting from a healing process in response to injury or long-term inflammation. Here are some key impacts of excessive fibrotic tissue:

- **Nerve damage:** If excessive fibrotic tissue compresses nerve cells, it could cause numbness, tingling sensations, or permanent nerve damage, resulting in loss of function and sensation. This can occur in conditions such as sciatica, carpal tunnel syndrome, and others.
- **Chronic Pain:** Fibrosis can lead to chronic pain, especially when it affects muscles, joints, or tissues involved in movement. Conditions such as Dupuytren's contracture, back pain, neck pain, sciatica, carpal tunnel syndrome, bursitis, tendonitis, plantar fasciitis, frozen shoulder, tension headaches, and trigger finger are examples where fibrosis can significantly contribute to discomfort and mobility issues.
- **Mobility Issues**: In muscles, tendons, and ligaments, fibrosis can restrict movement, leading to stiffness and pain. Typically, our muscles behave like a rubber band, stretching and elongating as they contract and relax. However, when fibrotic tissue is present in the muscle, it acts like a knot that limits muscle contraction, reduces range of motion, and causes pain.
- **Reduced Functionality**: Fibrotic tissue is less flexible than normal tissue, which can lead to impaired function of the affected organ or area. For example, in the lungs (as in pulmonary fibrosis), this can lead to difficulty breathing and decreased oxygen intake.
- **Organ Dysfunction**: In organs like the liver (cirrhosis), heart (cardiac fibrosis), and kidneys (renal fibrosis), excessive fibrotic tissue can disrupt normal function. This can result in a significant decrease in the organ's ability to perform its essential tasks, such as filtering blood, pumping blood, or metabolizing substances.
- **Increased Risk of Complications**: Fibrotic changes can increase the risk of further complications. For instance, liver cirrhosis, which involves fibrosis or scarring of the liver, can lead to complications such as portal hypertension and visceral bleeding.

- **Impaired Healing and Regeneration**: Excessive fibrosis can interfere with the normal healing process, as scar tissue can replace normal, healthy tissue, leading to prolonged or incomplete recovery.
- **Restricted Movement**: In cases where fibrosis affects the skin, muscles, or connective tissues (such as in scleroderma or after severe burns), it can lead to reduced mobility due to stiff and tightened tissues.
- **Aesthetic Concerns**: On the skin, fibrotic tissue can cause cosmetic concerns, especially if the scarring is extensive or occurs in highly visible areas.

### Ineffective Methods for Breaking Down Fibrotic Tissue

Fibrotic tissue, due to its thickness and hardness, requires firm mechanical force to break down. An understanding of the physiology of fibrosis shows that certain approaches are ineffective for breaking down fibrotic tissue. These include massage, foam rollers, manual therapy, Gua Sha, instrument-assisted soft tissue mobilization, stretching, and exercises.

1. **Foam rollers:** These approaches typically provide only superficial pressure on the tissue. In many cases, fibrotic tissue is located deep within muscles, such as in the hamstrings, quadriceps, and gluteus muscles, where it can be up to 2 inches deep. This renders foam rollers ineffective for reaching and treating these areas.
2. **Deep tissue massage:** Involves the therapist using their hands, knuckles, and/or elbows to reach deeper layers of muscle. However, due to the width and diameter of the therapist's knuckles and elbows, it is difficult to penetrate deep tissues and provide consistent forces necessary to break down deep fibrotic tissue
3. **Manual therapy:** Similar to massage, manual therapy often involves using the knuckles, elbows, or hands to reach deeper tissues. However, the relatively large diameter of the therapist's hands and elbows may limit their ability to penetrate deeply enough to effect physiological changes in fibrotic tissues located deep within muscles.
4. **Exercises and Stretching:** Do not exert sufficient mechanical force on fibrotic tissue to break it down; they simply cause movement in the muscle.

5. **Myofascial release:** Involves applying gentle, sustained pressure to the superficial connective tissue, which may not exert enough mechanical force to break down scar tissue or reach deeply enough to affect deep fibrosis.
6. **Gua Sha and Instrument-Assisted Soft Tissue Mobilization:** These techniques involve tools that might resemble rods or a butter knife, used to apply horizontal superficial force on the skin. Like manual therapy, they fail

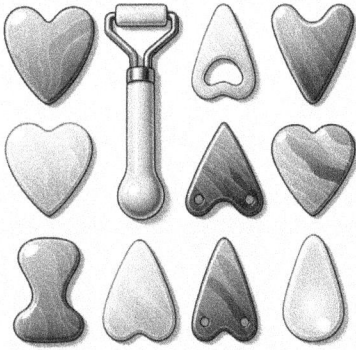

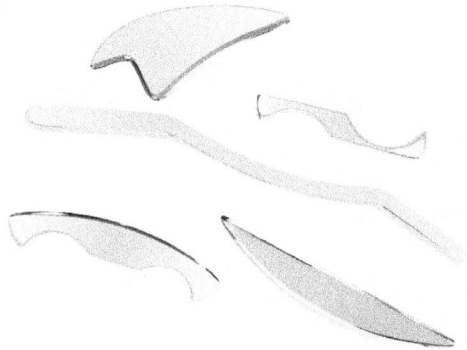

**Instrument Assisted Soft Tissue Mobilization (IASTM)**

**Gua Sha**

to penetrate deeply enough to alter fibrotic tissue effectively. This is like trying to unscrew a deep-set screw in a car with a screwdriver that is too short; it simply cannot reach deep enough to be effective.

## The Solution

Analyzing and testing current approaches that claim to break down fibrotic tissue led me to realize that it is physiologically impossible to effectively target both superficial and deep fibrotic tissue with these methods. This realization was the turning point that inspired the invention of ergonomically designed ASTR instruments. These instruments are specifically created to address both superficial and deep fibrotic tissue, capable of penetrating up to 2 inches deep to break down adhesions.

## 5. Fibrotic Tissue

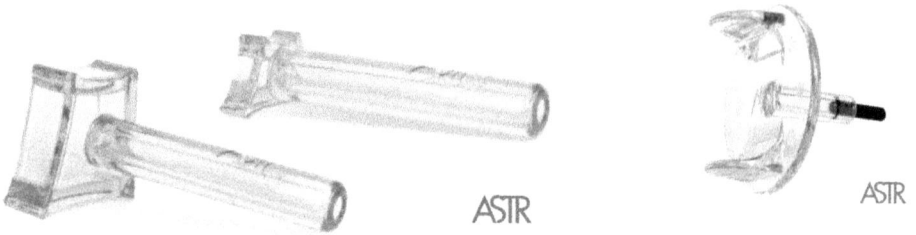

## Conclusion

In chronic back pain conditions, the affected areas of the body often become trapped in a persistent cycle of inflammation and tissue proliferation, preventing proper healing. This ongoing cycle leads to heightened inflammation, fibrosis, muscle spasms, and severe fascial restrictions, which contribute to the intensity and persistence of back pain. Nutritional deficiencies in essential vitamins and minerals can further hinder the body's ability to progress to the final stage of healing, keeping it locked in this disruptive pattern. Additionally, excessive fibrosis and fascial tightness can worsen the condition, making it even more difficult to break free from the cycle of chronic back pain.

## 6. Fascial Restrictions

## Myofascial Restrictions and Their Role in Back Pain

Myofascial restrictions, particularly the presence of myofascial trigger points (MTrPs), have been implicated in the development and persistence of chronic back pain. MTrPs are hyperirritable spots within taut bands of skeletal muscle fibers that can elicit local and referred pain upon palpation. Research has shown a high prevalence of active MTrPs in individuals with chronic low back pain, particularly in the lumbar and thoracic musculature (Fernández-de-Las-Peñas et al., 2018). A study conducted in a primary care setting found that approximately 30% of patients with musculoskeletal pain exhibited myofascial pain syndrome, with the back being the most frequently affected area (Gerwin et al., 2020). These findings suggest a strong association between myofascial dysfunction and back pain, highlighting the need for targeted interventions to address these restrictions.

The presence of MTrPs contributes to chronic back pain by increasing muscle tenderness and sensitizing central pain pathways, leading to prolonged discomfort and limited mobility. Research indicates that chronic activation of MTrPs can lead to peripheral and central sensitization, further lowering the pain threshold and exacerbating musculoskeletal dysfunction (Ge et al., 2020). Moreover, increased muscle tension due to fascial restrictions in the thoracolumbar fascia has been shown to impair movement and contribute to back pain persistence (Wilke et al., 2017). These findings emphasize the importance of addressing myofascial dysfunction as a critical component of effective back pain management.

The fascial system, an integral component of the body's connective tissue network, plays a crucial role in supporting and connecting all bodily structures. Here's a comprehensive overview of the fascial system:

## What is Fascia?

Next time you buy meat, look for the white filaments in it; those are the fascia layers. Fascia is a dense, tough tissue that extends throughout the body in a three-dimensional web from head to toe. It surrounds and interpenetrates every muscle, bone, nerve, blood vessel, and organ. Fascia is primarily made up of collagen fibers, which provide it with both flexibility and strength. Fascia is a

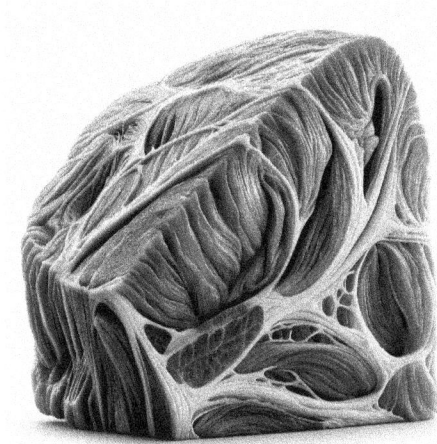

The white filaments in the meat are the fascia layers

complex network of connective tissue that extends throughout the body and plays a crucial role in supporting and protecting bodily structures.

## Key Attributes of the Fascial System

The fascia system, a continuous network of connective tissue that envelops and interconnects every structure in the body, plays a critical role in maintaining overall health and physical integrity. Here are the key attributes of the fascial system:

### 1. Ubiquity and Continuity

- Fascia is present throughout the entire body. It wraps around and interconnects muscles, bones, organs, nerves, and blood vessels, forming a seamless web that extends from head to toe. This continuity is crucial for the integration and coordination of bodily structures and functions.

### 2. Structural Support and Protection

- Fascia provides a framework that supports the body's structures. It helps maintain the position of organs, enables the transmission of muscular force, and protects internal structures from physical trauma.

### 3. Flexibility and Elasticity

- Despite its strength, fascia is also highly flexible and elastic. This allows it to stretch and move without restriction, accommodating movements of muscles and joints while returning to its original shape.

### 4. Sensory Role
- Fascia is richly innervated with nerve endings, making it an important sensory organ. These nerves are responsible for proprioception (the sense of body position and movement) and the perception of pain. This sensory role is essential for maintaining posture and physical coordination.

### 5. Fluid Transport
- The fascial network plays a role in the circulation of fluids throughout the body, including blood and lymphatic fluid. It facilitates the transport of nutrients and waste products to and from cells.

### 6. Metabolic Function
- Fascia can store energy in the form of fat and water, and it also provides pathways for inflammation and healing. The extracellular matrix within the fascia contains cells that can respond to and influence metabolic processes.

### 7. Adaptability
- Fascia is highly adaptable and responsive to physical and emotional stimuli. Chronic stress, injury, or poor postural habits can lead to changes in the fascial structures, sometimes leading to restrictions and pain.

### 8. Pathway for Force Transmission
- Fascia transmits mechanical tension generated by muscle activity or external forces across the body. This distribution of force helps in reducing local stress on muscles and joints and enhances overall movement efficiency.

### 9. Compartmentalization
- Through deeper layers, such as the deep fascia, it compartmentalizes sections of the body, segregating groups of muscles and other structures into functional units. This compartmentalization aids in organizing the body architecturally and facilitates effective movement and function.

These attributes illustrate why the fascial system is integral not only to movement and stability but also to the general health and well-being of the body. Understanding and addressing fascial health is crucial in sports, rehabilitation, and general physical maintenance.

## Layers of the Fascial System

There are several distinct layers of fascia, each with its specific function and characteristics. Understanding these layers helps in appreciating the complexity of human anatomy and the integration of bodily functions. Here's a detailed explanation of the different fascia layers:

1. **Superficial Fascia (Subcutaneous Tissue)**
   - **Location**: The superficial fascia layer is like a Spider-Man suit covering the whole body. Just below the skin, above the deeper layers of fascia.This layer separates the skin from the musculoskeletal system, allowing for normal sliding between the muscles and skin.
   - **Composition**: Consists of loose connective tissue and fat. This layer varies in thickness across different parts of the body and from person to person. Many nerve fibers are observed, and in some regions, the superficial fascia splits, forming specialized compartments. The collagen fibers are arranged irregularly. It consists of different layers that can slide over one another. The superficial fascia layer consists of two to three layers on top of each other
   - **Functions**: Acts as a water storage medium, provides insulation and padding, and allows the skin to move freely over underlying structures. It also serves as a conduit for nerves and blood vessels as they pass to and from the skin.

2. **Deep Fascia**
   - **Location**: Surrounds and infuses with muscles, bones, nerves, and blood vessels to the level of the dermis.
   - **Composition**: Denser than superficial fascia, this layer is made of tightly packed collagen fibers running in a parallel arrangement. It forms a fibrous sheath that encloses muscles and divides them into groups. Each subdivision of the deep fascia layer consists of two to three layers on top of each other.
   - **Functions**: Provides an extensive area for muscle attachment, enhances force transmission across muscles, and maintains structural integrity. The

# Musclar Fascia Layers

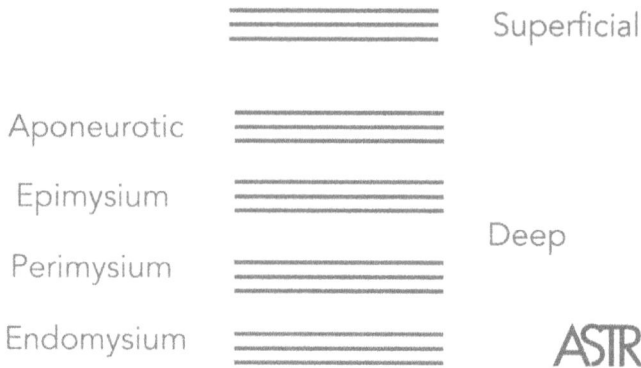

| | |
|---|---|
| | Superficial |
| Aponeurotic | |
| Epimysium | |
| | Deep |
| Perimysium | |
| Endomysium | |

ASTR

deep fascia also separates different functional areas of muscles, allowing them to operate independently.

**Division of Deep Fascia:**

- **Aponeurotic Fascia:** Surrounds groups of muscles. It consists of 2 or 3 layers of unidirectional collagen fibers, with each layer separated by loose connective tissue. Composed of 80% collagen fibers and only 1% elastic fibers. This fascia helps keep a group of muscles in place or serves as the insertion point for a broad muscle.
- **Epimysial Fascia:** Surrounds the entire muscle. It is formed of type I and III collagen and is specific to each muscle. It contains approximately 15% elastic fibers. The epimysium is free to glide due to being separated from the aponeurotic fascia by an external layer of loose connective tissue. It is thinner than the aponeurotic fascia and is also separated from the perimysial fascia by an internal layer of loose connective tissue. Multiple septa detach from the epimysium and insert into both the overlying aponeurotic fascia and the underlying perimysial fascia.
- **Perimysial Fascia:** Surrounds bundles of muscle fibers within a muscle. It consists of connective tissue that penetrates the muscle to support and

separate muscle fiber bundles (fascicles). This fascia provides the pathway for nerves and blood vessels to reach individual muscle fibers.
- **Endomysial Fascia:** Surrounds individual muscle fibers. It is a thin layer of connective tissue that supports capillaries and nerve fibers. The endomysium plays a crucial role in the transfer of force from the muscle fibers to the tendons.

3.   **Visceral Fascia (Subserous Fascia)**
- **Location**: Surrounds organs within the cavities of the body, such as the thoracic and abdominal cavities.
- **Composition**: Thinner and more delicate than deep fascia, and often contains a larger amount of elastic fibers to accommodate the movement and expansion of organs.
- **Functions**: The fascia holds organs in place and provides them with structural support. It also creates compartments within the body that can help limit the spread of infections or malignancies.

Each layer of fascia is integral to the functional architecture of the body, providing both structural support and flexibility. Problems in any layer of the fascia can lead to pain, reduced function, and mobility issues, highlighting the importance of this connective tissue system in overall health and well-being.

## Functions of the Fascial System

The fascial system has several crucial functions:
1.   **Support and Structure**: Fascia provides a supportive and stabilizing framework for all body structures. It holds organs in place and ensures that muscles and other structures maintain their proper alignment.
2.   **Force Transmission**: Through its tensile strength and structural continuity, fascia transmits mechanical loads and muscle forces efficiently across the body. This helps in maintaining balance and coordination during movement.
3.   **Protection**: Fascia acts as a protective layer over muscles and organs, cushioning them and reducing the impact of external forces.

4. **Separation and Compartmentalization**: By forming natural divisions between muscles and organs, fascia allows different body structures to slide smoothly over each other, facilitating efficient movement.

## Fascial restrictions

Fascia restrictions, often simply referred to as fascial restrictions, occur when the fascia, the connective tissue that surrounds and supports all structures within the body, becomes tight, stiff, or forms adhesions. These restrictions can significantly impact the body's mobility, flexibility, and function. Here's an in-depth look at fascia restrictions:

Fascial restrictions refer to the tightening or stiffening of the fascia, the connective tissue that surrounds and supports muscles, bones, nerves, and organs throughout the body. Fascia is supposed to be flexible and able to stretch as you move. However, due to various factors such as injury, surgery, inflammation, poor posture, or lack of activity, the fascia can become restricted. When fascial restrictions occur, they can limit mobility and cause pain, discomfort, or decreased range of motion. These restrictions can have a cascading effect on the body, potentially affecting overall biomechanical efficiency and leading to compensations in movement, which in turn might cause further discomfort or injury.

### Fascia Adhesion
Fascia adhesion occurs when the fascia, a thin layer of connective tissue that surrounds muscles, organs, and other structures, sticks to itself or to other tissues. This can restrict movement and cause pain.

### Fascia Fibrosis

Fascia fibrosis is the thickening and stiffening of the fascia due to excessive collagen deposition, often as a response to chronic inflammation or injury. This condition is more severe than simple adhesions and can significantly impair function.

### Causes of Fascia Restrictions
Fascia restrictions can arise from a variety of factors:

- **Injury**: Trauma from accidents or surgeries can lead to inflammation and subsequent fibrosis (scar tissue), which restricts the normal elasticity of fascia.
- **Repetitive Stress**: Repetitive activities or overuse injuries can lead to chronic inflammation and fibrotic changes in the fascia.
- **Poor Posture**: Prolonged poor posture can cause the fascia to adapt in maladaptive ways, leading to tension and restrictions.
- **Inactivity**: Lack of movement can cause fascia to become dehydrated and less pliable, making it prone to stiffness and adhesions.
- **Inflammatory Responses**: Systemic inflammation, as seen in various autoimmune disorders, can also affect the fascial system, making it less flexible.

## Symptoms of Fascia Restrictions

The presence of fascial restrictions can manifest in various symptoms:

- **Reduced Mobility**: Stiffness and limited range of motion in joints.
- **Pain**: Chronic pain is often described as a deep, aching, or band-like pain that may increase with movement or touch.
- **Tension**: A feeling of tightness in the muscles and surrounding areas.
- **Sensory Changes**: Some individuals might experience tingling or numbness due to the pressure on nerves by tight fascia.
- **Misalignment**: Fascial restrictions can pull the body out of alignment, affecting posture and leading to compensatory patterns elsewhere in the body.

### Ineffective Methods for Releasing Fascial Restrictions

The fascia system is so complex that it requires targeted tools to release each restricted layer. Random hand movements without gripping the fascia layer will not mobilize it to release the adhesions that cause the layers to stick together and prevent them from gliding freely on top of each other. An understanding of the physiology of the fascia system shows that certain approaches are ineffective for releasing it, including massage, foam rollers, manual therapy, Gua Sha, instrument-assisted soft tissue mobilization, stretching, and exercises.

1. **Foam rollers:** Typically, they provide only superficial pressure on the tissue. Gliding the foam roller over just the superficial layer will not release the

adhesions, and the foam roller will not apply enough deep pressure to release the epimysium, perimysium, and endomysium layers.

2. **Deep tissue massage:** Involves the therapist using their hands, knuckles, and/or elbows to reach deeper layers of muscle. However, due to the width and diameter of the therapist's knuckles and elbows, it is difficult to penetrate deep tissues and provide the consistent gripping forces necessary to release deep fascia adhesions.

3. **Manual therapy:** Similar to massage, it often involves using the knuckles, elbows, or hands to reach deeper tissues. However, the relatively large diameter of the therapist's hands and elbows may limit their ability to penetrate deeply enough to effect physiological changes in fascia layers located deep within muscles. Additionally, it is very difficult for the hand to grip deep fascia layers to release them.

4. **Exercises and stretching:** Do not exert sufficient mechanical force on fascia layers to cause adhesion release; they simply cause movement in the muscle.

5. **Myofascial release:** This involves applying gentle, sustained pressure to the superficial connective tissue, which addresses the superficial fascia layer but does not go deep enough to release the aponeurotic, epimysium,

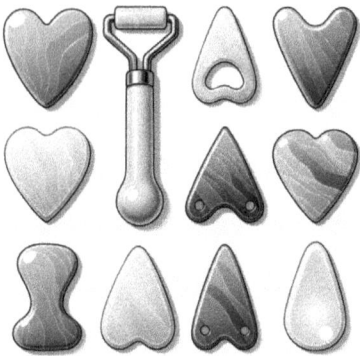

Gua Sha

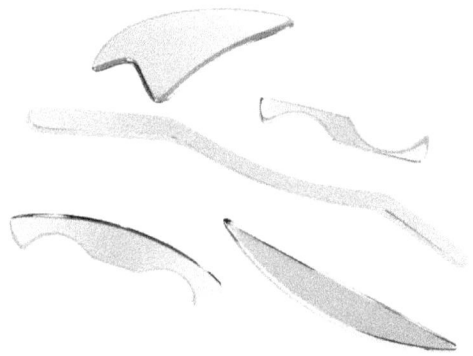

Instrument Assisted Soft Tissue Mobilization (IASTM)

perimysium, and endomysium fascia layers.

6. **Gua Sha and Instrument-Assisted Soft Tissue Mobilization:** These techniques involve tools that might resemble rods or a butter knife, used to apply horizontal superficial force on the skin. Like manual therapy, they fail

to penetrate deeply enough to alter the fascia system and are unable to grip the fascia layers to release them. This is like trying to unscrew a deep-set screw in a car with a screwdriver that is too short; it simply cannot reach deep enough to be effective.

**The Solution**

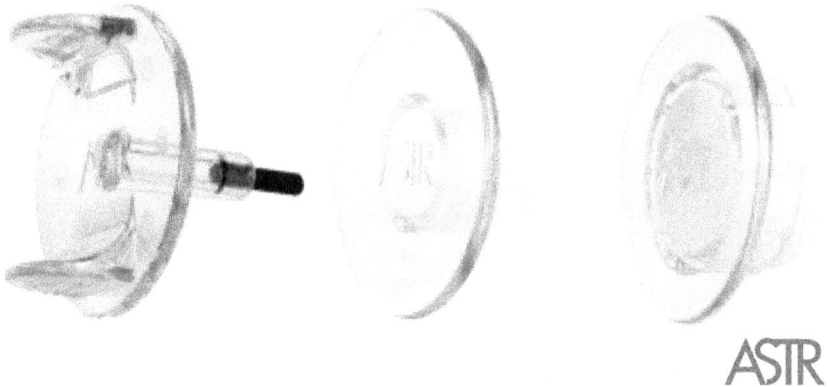

Analyzing and testing current approaches that claim to provide myofascial release led me to realize that it is physiologically impossible to effectively target both superficial and deep fascia layers with these methods. This realization was the turning point that inspired the invention of ergonomically designed ASTR instruments. These instruments are specifically created to address superficial fascia, aponeurotic fascia, epimysium, perimysium, and endomysium layers. They are capable of penetrating up to 2 inches deep to release the epimysium, perimysium, and endomysium.

**Conclusion**

In chronic back pain conditions, the body often becomes trapped in a continuous cycle of inflammation and tissue proliferation, preventing proper healing. This ongoing process leads to widespread inflammation, fibrosis, muscle spasms, and severe fascial restrictions, all of which contribute to the persistence and intensity of back pain. Deficiencies in essential vitamins and minerals can further disrupt the body's ability to progress to the final stage of healing, keeping it locked in this dysfunctional pattern. Additionally, excessive fibrosis and fascial tension can amplify the condition, making it even more difficult to break free from the cycle of chronic back pain.

This persistent cycle highlights the limitations of the biomedical model in effectively treating chronic back pain, as it primarily focuses on symptom management rather than addressing the root causes such as fibrotic tissue, fascial restrictions, and underlying hormonal and nutritional imbalances. Without a comprehensive, holistic approach, the body remains stuck in this repetitive pattern, preventing true recovery.

# 7. Behavior Modification

## Behavior Modification for Managing Back Pain

Behavior modification is a therapeutic approach used to replace undesirable behaviors with more beneficial ones through the systematic application of learning principles and techniques. Rooted in the theories of operant conditioning developed by John B. Watson and B.F. Skinner, behavior modification operates on the premise that behaviors can be learned and unlearned based on the consequences they produce.

This approach can be highly effective in managing chronic back pain by addressing lifestyle habits, environmental factors, and stressors that contribute to pain persistence and severity. Many back pain triggers, such as poor posture, lack of movement, stress responses, and improper lifting techniques, develop over time. By applying systematic techniques, individuals can adopt healthier behaviors that reduce back pain intensity and frequency.

### Identifying Contributing Behaviors

The first step in behavior modification is identifying and clearly defining behaviors that contribute to chronic back pain. These may include:

- **Poor Postural Habits:** Forward head posture, prolonged sitting, and improper workplace ergonomics that lead to muscular tension and spinal misalignment (Wang et al., 2021).
- **Sedentary Lifestyle:** Prolonged inactivity and lack of movement, which can weaken core and back muscles, leading to instability and pain (Smith et al., 2019).
- **Stress-Related Behaviors:** Chronic stress, poor stress management, and increased muscle tension contributing to back pain flare-ups (Zhu et al., 2022).
- **Improper Lifting Techniques:** Incorrect lifting mechanics that place excessive strain on the lower back, increasing the risk of injury (Marras et al., 2018).

### Setting Goals for Behavior Modification

Setting SMART goals (Specific, Measurable, Achievable, Relevant, and Time-bound) helps individuals modify behaviors effectively. Examples include:

- **Improve posture awareness** by using ergonomic chairs and taking posture breaks every 30 minutes for four weeks.
- **Increase daily movement** by incorporating five-minute mobility exercises every two hours.
- **Manage stress-related behaviors** by practicing deep breathing or mindfulness exercises for five minutes, three times a day.

## Techniques for Behavior Modification

Several techniques can be employed to modify behaviors linked to chronic back pain:

- **Education and Awareness:** Many individuals unknowingly engage in behaviors that worsen back pain. Learning about proper posture, movement mechanics, and pain triggers can empower individuals to make informed changes (McGill, 2016).
- **Self-Monitoring:** Tracking pain patterns, daily activities, and triggers using a back pain journal or mobile app can help identify correlations and adjust behaviors accordingly (Kongsted et al., 2021).
- **Positive Reinforcement:** Rewarding positive behaviors, such as maintaining an exercise routine or improving workplace ergonomics, encourages long-term adherence.
- **Cueing and Prompting:** Using reminders, alarms, or habit-tracking apps to prompt posture corrections, hydration, and stretching exercises reinforces healthy habits.
- **Feedback:** Seeking input from a healthcare provider, or physical therapist can provide accountability and necessary adjustments to behavior modification strategies.
- **Modeling:** Observing others successfully managing back pain through corrective exercises, stress management, and ergonomic changes can inspire individuals to implement similar strategies.

## Maintenance and Generalization

Once new behaviors are learned, they need to be maintained and applied across different situations. This includes:

- **Consistent Practice:** Continuing core strengthening exercises, maintaining proper posture, and applying stress management techniques even after symptoms improve.
- **Social Support:** Engaging family, friends, or coworkers to encourage and remind individuals about their back pain management strategies.
- **Environmental Adjustments:** Modify home and work environments to support behavioral changes, such as investing in an ergonomic workspace or ensuring proper sleep support with a high-quality mattress.

## Conclusion

Following the recommendations outlined in posture and behavior modification strategies can provide guidance on necessary lifestyle changes. For individuals experiencing persistent back pain despite behavioral adjustments, consulting a healthcare provider trained in behavioral therapy and ergonomics is advisable. Those with postural-related back pain may require ergonomic corrections and targeted exercises to address musculoskeletal imbalances. By addressing underlying habits and making sustainable modifications, individuals can take a proactive role in reducing back pain and improving overall well-being.

## Conclusion

# Conclusion

Healing from back pain requires a comprehensive approach that goes beyond simply managing symptoms. Throughout this book, we have explored seven natural strategies that address the root causes of chronic back pain, helping you break free from persistent discomfort and regain control over your health. By identifying inflammatory foods, balancing essential vitamins, minerals, and hormones, and correcting postural imbalances, you can support your body's natural healing process. Managing stress, addressing fibrotic tissue and fascial restrictions, and modifying harmful behaviors further enhance recovery and pain prevention.

One of the most critical aspects of this journey is ensuring that your body has the proper nutritional foundation to transition from chronic inflammation to full recovery. Deficiencies in essential vitamins, minerals, and hormones can prevent the body from properly regulating inflammation, repairing musculoskeletal tissues, and restoring structural balance. Many individuals with chronic back pain suffer from underlying deficiencies without realizing it, keeping them trapped in a cycle of pain, fatigue, and limited mobility. Research suggests that deficiencies in vitamin D, magnesium, and B vitamins are commonly associated with chronic musculoskeletal pain, including back pain (Gordon et al., 2020).

From my clinical experience, patients with chronic back pain typically exhibit at least three to six vitamin and mineral deficiencies. To optimize the healing process, it is essential to work with a clinical nutritionist who can assess nutritional balance through comprehensive lab testing. Identifying and correcting these deficiencies will enhance the body's ability to recover and improve the effectiveness of the other strategies presented in this book.

Each of the seven elements discussed plays a significant role in reducing back pain intensity and frequency. Addressing only one or two areas may provide partial relief, but achieving lasting improvement requires a multi-faceted approach. Identifying food triggers and eliminating pro-inflammatory foods can reduce unnecessary stress on the body, helping to prevent pain flare-ups. Maintaining proper posture and addressing musculoskeletal imbalances can further relieve tension and reduce spinal misalignment that contributes to back pain. Managing stress is crucial, as chronic stress leads to hormonal imbalances, nervous system overactivity, and muscle tension, all of which can exacerbate back pain symptoms (Zhu et al., 2022).

# Conclusion

Treating fibrotic tissue and fascial restrictions can improve circulation, reduce nerve compression, and promote soft tissue healing, all of which support long-term pain reduction. Behavior modification is equally important in changing habits and reinforcing positive lifestyle adjustments that prevent back pain from recurring.

By approaching back pain treatment with a holistic and personalized strategy, individuals can achieve sustainable relief and improved overall well-being. The process of healing takes time and commitment, but with the right knowledge and support, it is possible to regain control over your health. Taking proactive steps to address nutritional imbalances, lifestyle factors, and structural issues can transform how the body responds to pain and restore balance. Through consistent application of these principles, you can move beyond managing chronic back pain and toward a healthier, pain-free life.

# Recommended Resources

**How to Access Online Content**
1. Open the camera app on your smartphone.
2. Point the camera at the barcode.
3. A notification will appear with a link. Tap the notification to open the link in your browser.

1. Posture and Body Mechanics Training Videos

2. Case Studies and Recorded Live Treatment Videos

3. <u>Limited Time Offer</u>: FREE 30-minute Health Coach Consultation

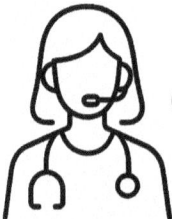

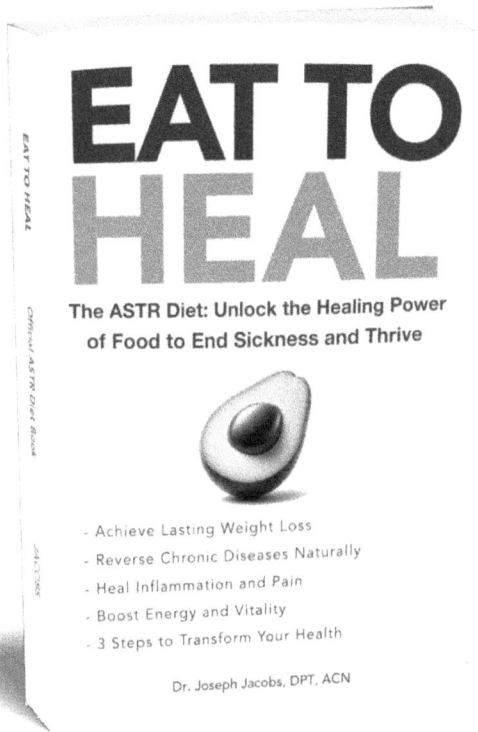

# EAT TO HEAL

## The ASTR Diet: Unlock the Healing Power of Food to End Sickness and Thrive

- Achieve Lasting Weight Loss
- Reverse Chronic Diseases Naturally
- Heal Inflammation and Pain
- Boost Energy and Vitality
- 3 Steps to Transform Your Health

Dr. Joseph Jacobs, DPT, ACN

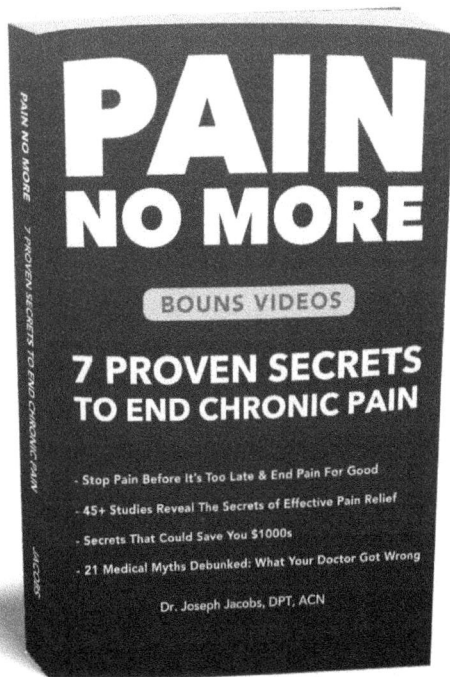

# PAIN NO MORE

BOUNS VIDEOS

## 7 PROVEN SECRETS TO END CHRONIC PAIN

- Stop Pain Before It's Too Late & End Pain For Good
- 45+ Studies Reveal The Secrets of Effective Pain Relief
- Secrets That Could Save You $1000s
- 21 Medical Myths Debunked: What Your Doctor Got Wrong

Dr. Joseph Jacobs, DPT, ACN

# BEATING
## MIGRAINES

**BONUS VIDEOS**

### 7 NATURAL SECRETS FOR
### LASTING RELIEF

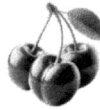

- End Migraines Naturally
- Clinically Proven Methods
- Treat the Root Cause, Not Symptoms
- Insights from a Doctor & Migraine Survivor
- Research-Backed Relief for Life

Dr. Joseph Jacobs, DPT, ACN

# BEATING
# ANXIETY
## &
## DEPRESSION

**BONUS VIDEOS**

### 14 NATURAL SECRETS TO
### A HAPPIER LIFE

- Conquer Anxiety & Depression Naturally
- Heal the Root Causes & Reclaim Your Life
- Created by a Doctor Who Conquered PTSD & Depression
- Science-Based Strategies for Lasting Change

Dr. Joseph Jacobs, DPT, ACN

# REVERSING
## HIGH BLOOD
## PRESSURE

### 7 NATURAL SECRETS TO SAFELY
### LOWER BLOOD PRESSURE

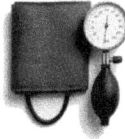

- Natural Solutions That Work
- Backed by Extensive Research
- Fix the Root Cause, Not Just the Numbers
- No Drugs, No Side Effects

Dr. Joseph Jacobs, DPT, ACN

# REVERSING
## DIABETES

### 10 NATURAL SECRETS TO REVERSE
### DIABETES WITHOUT DRUGS

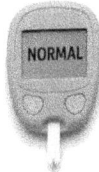

NORMAL

- Drug-Free, Side-Effect-Free, Science-Backed Healing
- Treat the Root Cause, Not Just the Symptoms
- Proven Natural Strategies That Get Results

Dr. Joseph Jacobs, DPT, ACN

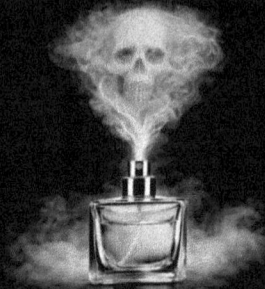

KILLED BY
FRAGRANCE

*How Synthetic Scents Make Us Sick*

- Exposed by peer-reviewed research
- Links everyday fragrance exposure to chronic disease
- Built on science, not opinion

Dr. Joseph Jacobs, DPT, ACN

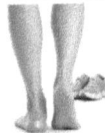

*Your*
SHOES
HURT YOU

Why Does Your Pain Keep Coming
Back and *How to Fix It*

BONUS VIDEOS

- Fix Your Feet. Fix Your Pain.
- Why Modern Shoes Create Chronic Pain
- Backed by Biomechanics and Clinical Research

Dr. Joseph Jacobs, DPT, ACN

103

# Glossary

**Acute Inflammation** - A short-term immune response to injury or infection, characterized by redness, swelling, heat, and pain.

**Ankylosing Spondylitis** - A type of inflammatory arthritis that affects the spine and can lead to spinal fusion, causing stiffness and chronic pain.

**Anti-Inflammatory Diet** - A nutritional approach that focuses on consuming foods that reduce inflammation and promote overall health, as outlined in the ASTR Diet.

**ASTR Diet** - A diet developed by Dr. Joseph Jacobs, emphasizing anti-inflammatory, sustainable, toxin-free, and restorative principles to support healing and wellness.

**ASTR Treatment** - A holistic treatment approach developed by Dr. Joseph Jacobs that integrates manual therapy, behavior modification, and nutritional support to address chronic pain.

**Behavior Modification** - The process of changing lifestyle habits, such as posture, diet, and movement patterns, to reduce chronic pain and promote long-term healing.

**Biomechanics** - The study of movement and the forces acting upon the body to improve function and reduce pain, particularly related to posture and musculoskeletal health.

**Chronic Fatigue** - A persistent state of physical and mental exhaustion that is not alleviated by rest and may be linked to chronic inflammation and nutrient deficiencies.

**Chronic Inflammation** - A prolonged and persistent inflammatory response that can contribute to various health conditions, including autoimmune diseases and chronic pain.

**Compression Fractures** - Fractures in the vertebrae that can cause severe back pain, often due to osteoporosis or traumatic injury.

**Connective Tissue** - A type of biological tissue that supports, binds, and connects other tissues and organs in the body, playing a key role in musculoskeletal health.

**Degenerative Disc Disease** - A condition in which the intervertebral discs deteriorate over time, leading to pain, stiffness, and reduced mobility.

**Detoxification** - The process of eliminating toxins from the body to improve health and restore balance, emphasized in the ASTR approach.

**Elimination Diet** - A dietary approach that removes certain foods to identify intolerances or sensitivities contributing to inflammation and chronic pain.

**Fascial Restriction** - Tightening of the fascia that can limit movement and contribute to chronic pain, often released through specialized manual therapy techniques.

**Fibrotic Tissue** - Excess connective tissue that develops due to injury, inflammation, or repetitive stress, often leading to restricted movement and pain.

**Failed Back Surgery Syndrome (FBSS)** - A condition in which patients continue to experience chronic pain following spinal surgery due to nerve damage, scar tissue, or unresolved issues.

**Herniated Disc** - A condition in which the soft inner portion of an intervertebral disc pushes through the outer layer, potentially compressing nearby nerves and causing pain.

**Holistic Healing** - An approach to health that considers the whole person—body, mind, and spirit—rather than just treating symptoms, as applied in the ASTR treatment model.

**Hormonal Imbalance** - Disruptions in hormone levels that can affect pain perception, inflammation, and musculoskeletal function, often addressed through dietary and lifestyle interventions.

# Glossary

**Inflammation** - The body's natural response to injury, infection, or irritants, which can be either acute or chronic and plays a role in pain conditions like sciatica and spinal stenosis.

**Intermittent Fasting** - A dietary strategy that alternates periods of eating and fasting to promote metabolic health and reduce inflammation, incorporated into the ASTR Diet.

**Lymphatic System** - A network of vessels and nodes that help remove waste, toxins, and excess fluids from the body while supporting immune function.

**Micronutrients** - Essential vitamins and minerals required in small amounts to support bodily functions and overall health, often deficient in individuals with chronic pain.

**Myofascial Release** - A manual therapy technique used to relieve tension in the fascia and improve mobility, often utilized in ASTR treatments.

**Neuropathy** - A condition involving nerve damage that can cause pain, numbness, and weakness, often linked to chronic inflammation and nutrient deficiencies.

**Nutrient Deficiency** - A lack of essential vitamins and minerals necessary for optimal bodily function, often contributing to chronic health conditions and back pain.

**Osteoarthritis** - A degenerative joint disease that leads to the breakdown of cartilage, causing pain, stiffness, and reduced mobility.

**Osteoporosis** - A condition characterized by weakened bones, increasing the risk of fractures, particularly in the spine.

**Piriformis Syndrome** - A neuromuscular disorder in which the piriformis muscle compresses the sciatic nerve, leading to pain and discomfort.

**Postural Imbalance** - Misalignment of the spine and body posture that contributes to back pain and muscular strain, commonly addressed in ASTR treatments.

**Proliferation Stage** - A phase of tissue healing in which new cells are generated, and inflammation is regulated to promote recovery, crucial in the back pain healing process.

**Radiculopathy** - A condition caused by compression or irritation of nerve roots in the spine, leading to pain, weakness, and numbness in the affected areas.

**Sciatica** - Pain caused by compression or irritation of the sciatic nerve, often due to a herniated disc, fibrotic tissue in the piriformis muscle, or spinal stenosis.

**Scoliosis** - An abnormal curvature of the spine that can cause pain and postural imbalances.

**Soft Tissue Mobilization** - A technique used to improve mobility and reduce pain by manipulating muscles, fascia, and other soft tissues, commonly used in ASTR treatments.

**Spinal Stenosis** - A condition characterized by the narrowing of the spinal canal, which can compress nerves and lead to pain, weakness, or numbness.

**Spondylolisthesis** - A condition where one vertebra slips forward over another, potentially causing instability and back pain.

**Stress Management** - Strategies such as mindfulness, relaxation techniques, and behavioral changes that help reduce stress-related muscle tension and inflammation.

**Tendonitis** - Inflammation of the tendons, which can contribute to musculoskeletal pain and dysfunction.

**Toxin-Free Nutrition** - An approach to eating that avoids harmful chemicals, additives, and processed foods to support health and healing, fundamental to the ASTR Diet.

**Trigger Points** - Hyperirritable spots in muscle tissue that can cause pain and referred discomfort in other areas of the body, often treated with myofascial release.

**Vitamin and Mineral Supplementation** - The use of dietary supplements to address deficiencies and support overall health, particularly in cases of chronic back pain.

# References

1. Bogduk N. On the definitions and physiology of back pain, referred pain, and radicular pain. Pain. 2009;147(1-3):17-19. pubmed.ncbi.nlm.nih.gov
2. Adams MA, Bogduk N, Burton K, Dolan P. The Biomechanics of Back Pain. 3rd ed. Churchill Livingstone; 2012. en.wikipedia.org
3. Mayo Clinic Staff. Back pain - Symptoms and causes. Mayo Clinic. Published February 2023. mayoclinic.org
4. National Institute of Neurological Disorders and Stroke. Low Back Pain Fact Sheet. NINDS. Published March 2020.
5. Physiopedia. Lumbosacral Biomechanics. Physiopedia. physio-pedia.com+1physio-pedia.com+1
6. Medscape. Mechanical Low Back Pain. Medscape Reference. Published October 2022. emedicine.medscape.com
7. MDPI. Mechanisms behind the Development of Chronic Low Back Pain. MDPI. Published January 2023. mdpi.com
8. StatPearls. Back Pain. NCBI Bookshelf. Published 2022. ncbi.nlm.nih.gov
9. Physiopedia. Low Back Pain. Physiopedia. physio-pedia.com
10. BMC Musculoskeletal Disorders. Hip biomechanics in patients with low back pain, what do we know. BMC Musculoskeletal Disorders. Published 2023
11. National Center for Health Statistics. Back, Lower Limb, and Upper Limb Pain Among U.S. Adults, 2019. Centers for Disease Control and Prevention. https://www.cdc.gov/nchs/products/databriefs/db415.htm. Published November 2020.
12. World Health Organization. Low back pain. https://www.who.int/news-room/fact-sheets/detail/low-back-pain. Published March 2022.
13. Institute for Health Metrics and Evaluation. New study shows low back pain is the leading cause of disability globally. https://www.healthdata.org/news-events/newsroom/news-releases/lancet-new-study-shows-low-back-pain-leading-cause-disability. Published June 2023.
14. National Institute of Neurological Disorders and Stroke. Low Back Pain Fact Sheet. https://www.ninds.nih.gov/sites/default/files/migrate-documents/low_back_pain_20-ns-5161_march_2020_508c.pdf. Published March 2020.\
15. Merck Manual. Low Back Pain - Bone, Joint, and Muscle Disorders. https://www.merckmanuals.com/home/bone-joint-and-muscle-disorders/low-back-and-neck-pain/low-back-pain. Published November 2023.
16. American Society of Anesthesiologists. Back Pain - Causes & Treatment. https://madeforthismoment.asahq.org/pain-management/types-of-pain/back-pain/. Published February 2023.
17. Thomson S. Failed back surgery syndrome – definition, epidemiology and demographics. *Br J Pain*. 2013;7(1):56-59. doi:10.1177/2049463713506688. Available from: https://www.ncbi.nlm.nih.gov/pmc/articles/PMC4590156/
18. Basiaga B, Kłosek M, Kocjan G, et al. Failed back surgery syndrome (FBSS) – etiology, diagnosis and treatment. Archiv Euromedica. 2024;14(3):5-10.
19. Garg B, Meena D, Sharma V, Sinha S. Failed back surgery syndrome: a review article. BMC Musculoskeletal Disorders. 2022;23(1):456.
20. Henschke N, Maher CG, Refshauge KM, et al. Prevalence of and factors associated with failed back surgery syndrome: A retrospective cohort study. Spine (Phila Pa 1976). 2021;46(2):E88-E95.
21. Kumar K, Taylor RS, Jacques L, et al. Spinal cord stimulation versus conventional medical management for neuropathic pain: A multicentre randomised controlled trial in patients with failed back surgery syndrome. Pain. 2007;132(1-2):179-88.

# References

22. Manchikanti L, Benyamin RM, Falco FJ, et al. A critical appraisal of the prevalence of failed back surgery syndrome in the United States. Pain Physician. 2011;14(2):E69-79.
23. Schultz DM, McKean J, Norvell DC, et al. Reoperation rates and predictors following spinal fusion: A systematic review and meta-analysis. Neurosurgery. 2021;88(4):711-724.
24. Thapa P, Euasobhon P, Maneesai P, et al. Failed back surgery syndrome—terminology, etiology, prevention, and treatment: A review. Yeungnam Univ J Med. 2023;40(1):8-15.
25. Thapa P, Euasobhon P, Maneesai P, et al. Failed back surgery syndrome—terminology, etiology, prevention, and treatment: a review. *Yeungnam Univ J Med*. 2023;40(1):8-15.
26. Henschke N, Maher CG, Refshauge KM, et al. Prevalence of and factors associated with failed back surgery syndrome: A retrospective cohort study. *Spine (Phila Pa 1976)*. 2021;46(2):E88-E95.
27. Schultz DM, McKean J, Norvell DC, et al. Reoperation rates and predictors following spinal fusion: A systematic review and meta-analysis. *Neurosurgery*. 2021;88(4):711-724.
28. Steiner TJ, Stovner LJ. Global epidemiology of chronic musculoskeletal pain. *J Neurol Sci*. 2023;44(1):56-64.
29. Burch R, Rizzoli P, Loder E. The prevalence and impact of chronic back pain in the United States: A population-based study. *Pain Med*. 2022;23(4):789-795.
30. Ashina M, Katsarava Z, Do TP, et al. Global burden and risk factors of chronic back pain: A systematic review. *Lancet Neurol*. 2021;20(9):678-692.
31. Shin, D., Lee, K. W., Brann, L., Shivappa, N., & Hébert, J. R. (2022). Pro-inflammatory diet associated with low back pain in adults aged 50 years and older: Data from the National Health and Nutrition Examination Survey. *Applied Nursing Research*, 64, 151589. https://doi.org/10.1016/j.apnr.2022.151589
32. Shin, C. M., Lee, D. H., Seo, A. Y., Kim, N., & Kim, K. M. (2022). Proinflammatory dietary intake relates to pain sensitivity in chronic low back pain patients: A case-control study. *Pain*, 163(12), 2336-2345. https://doi.org/10.1097/j.pain.0000000000002638
33. Glover, T. L., Goodin, B. R., King, C. D., & Sibille, K. T. (2021). Vitamin D deficiency and chronic pain: Mechanisms, assessment, and potential clinical implications. *Pain Medicine, 22*(3), 458-471.
34. Jahromi, S. R., Togha, M., & Ghorbani, Z. (2019). The role of magnesium deficiency in chronic pain and musculoskeletal disorders. *Neurological Research, 41*(5), 377-384.
35. Martin, V. T., & Behbehani, M. M. (2006). Ovarian hormones and migraine headache: Understanding mechanisms and pathogenesis. *Headache, 46*(3), 365-386.
36. Yabanlı, A., & Özer, E. (2022). The impact of zinc deficiency on chronic pain syndromes. *Pain Research and Management, 2022*, 1-7.
37. Yip, C. H., Chiu, T. T., & Poon, A. T. (2008). The relationship between head posture and severity and disability of patients with neck pain. *Manual Therapy, 13*(2), 148-154.
38. Jun, H. J., Lee, J., & Kim, J. (2017). The association between posture and musculoskeletal pain among Korean adults: A nationwide cross-sectional study. *Journal of Orthopaedic & Sports Physical Therapy, 47*(9), 655-664
39. American Chiropractic Association. (2021). *Posture and back pain: What you need to know*. Retrieved from https://www.acatoday.org
40. American Psychological Association. (2021). Stress and chronic pain: The psychological connection. *APA Health Bulletin*. Retrieved from https://www.apa.org
41. Borsook, D., Maleki, N., Becerra, L., & McEwen, B. (2012). Understanding stress and chronic pain: A neural perspective. *Neuroscience & Biobehavioral Reviews, 36*(1), 1-10.
42. Davis, M., Quartana, P., & Burns, J. (2018). The role of stress fluctuations in the onset of back pain episodes. *Pain Medicine, 19*(4), 789-797.

# References

43. Kim, J. (2024). Cortisol and chronic pain: Examining the impact of HPA axis dysfunction on musculoskeletal disorders. *Journal of Pain Research, 17*(2), 211-225.

44. Sauro, K. M., & Becker, W. J. (2009). The stress-pain connection: Understanding mechanisms and management strategies. *Pain Research and Management, 14*(3), 221-230.

45. van der Meulen, M., Leijon, M., & Nyberg, L. (2020). Stress and musculoskeletal pain: The impact of psychological factors on back pain prevalence. *European Journal of Pain, 24*(6), 1125-1137.

46. Langevin HM, Sherman KJ, Pathria MN. Beyond fascia: Exploring the role of tissue fibrosis in chronic low back pain. *Pain Med.* 2011;12(3):364-377. doi:10.1111/j.1526-4637.2011.01086.x

47. Wilke J, Macchi V, De Caro R, Stecco C. Fascia and chronic pain: Current state and implications for treatment. *J Anat.*2017;231(1):147-157. doi:10.1111/joa.12633

48. Schilder A, Hoheisel U, Mense S. The impact of fascia on musculoskeletal pain: A systematic review. *Pain Res Manag.*2018;2018:5477156. doi:10.1155/2018/5477156

49. Bennett G, Seruya M, Fernandes J, et al. Epidural fibrosis and its relationship to failed back surgery syndrome. *Neurosurg Clin N Am.* 2018;29(4):459-468. doi:10.1016/j.nec.2018.07.007

50. Bosscher HA, Heavner JE. Incidence and severity of epidural fibrosis after back surgery: An analysis of the literature. *Pain Pract.* 2010;10(4):277-282. doi:10.1111/j.1533-2500.2010.00375.x

51. Zhao L, Yang F, Du L, et al. Intervertebral disc fibrosis and its role in chronic low back pain: Mechanisms and therapeutic targets. *J Orthop Res.* 2021;39(5):963-973. doi:10.1002/jor.24767

52. Kongsted A, Ris I, Kjaer P, Hartvigsen J. Self-management of back pain: How can we promote and evaluate improvements? *Pain Reports.* 2021;6(1):e873. doi:10.1097/PR9.0000000000000873

53. Marras WS, Ferguson SA, Burr D, Davis KG, Gupta P. Functional impairment and spine loading after repetitive lifting exertions. *Spine J.* 2018;18(5):805-813. doi:10.1016/j.spinee.2017.09.010

54. McGill SM. Low Back Disorders: Evidence-Based Prevention and Rehabilitation. 3rd ed. Human Kinetics; 2016.

55. Smith JA, Hoy DG, Cross M, Vos T, Naghavi M, Buchbinder R. Global prevalence of low back pain: A systematic review and meta-analysis. *Arthritis Rheumatol.* 2019;71(6): 1048-1055. doi:10.1002/art.40815

56. Wang X, Straker L, O'Sullivan P, Smith A. The impact of prolonged sitting on the musculoskeletal system and the effectiveness of interventions: A systematic review. *Ergonomics.* 2021;64(3):309-327. doi:10.1080/00140139.2020.1862312

57. Zhu W, Zeng N, Wang N, Chen C. The relationship between stress and chronic back pain: A systematic review and meta-analysis. *J Psychosom Res.* 2022;152:110672. doi:10.1016/j.jpsychores.2021.110672

58. Gordon W, Hoffman L, Bonner D. Vitamin D and chronic musculoskeletal pain: A review of current research. *Clin J Pain.* 2020;36(7):589-597. doi:10.1097/AJP.0000000000000846

59. Zhu W, Zeng N, Wang N, Chen C. The relationship between stress and chronic back pain: A systematic review and meta-analysis. *J Psychosom Res.* 2022;152:110672. doi:10.1016/j.jpsychores.2021.110672

60. Health.com. Can your morning coffee be causing inflammation? Here's what research says. 2024. Available from: https://www.health.com/can-your-morning-coffee-be-causing-inflammation-8764006

61. Health.com. What happens to your body when you eat fewer ultra-processed foods. 2024. Available from: https://www.health.com/what-happens-when-you-eat-fewer-ultra-processed-foods-11689787

# References

62. Physiotattva. 10 best foods to avoid if you suffer from chronic pain. 2024. Available from: https://www.physiotattva.com/blog/10-best-foods-to-avoid-if-you-suffer-from-chronic-pain

63. The Scottish Sun. Bowel doctor reveals things you should never do. 2024. Available from: https://www.thescottishsun.co.uk/health/14470574/bowel-doctor-things-never-risk-cancer-constipation

64. Mansouri, M., Pasdar, Y., Nachvak, S. M., Darbandi, M., Moradi, S., Mostafai, R., & Naja, F. (2022). Major dietary patterns in relation to chronic low back pain. *BMC Musculoskeletal Disorders, 23*(1), 393. https://doi.org/10.1186/s12891-022-05363-9

65. Mahan, L. K., & Escott-Stump, S. (2008). *Krause's Food & Nutrition Therapy* (12th ed.). Saunders Elsevier.

66. Yadav, D., & Lowenfels, A. B. (2013). The epidemiology of pancreatitis and pancreatic cancer. *Gastroenterology, 144*(6), 1252-1261. https://doi.org/10.1053/j.gastro.2013.01.068

67. Shiri, R., Falah-Hassani, K., & Heliövaara, M. (2013). Coffee, tea, caffeine consumption, and risk of low back pain: a systematic review and meta-analysis. *Nutrition Journal, 12*, 89. https://doi.org/10.1186/1475-2891-12-89

68. Joseph J, Madison S, Tiffany J, Henry H, Mario V, et al . Evaluating the Effectiveness of Treatment Options for Pain: Literature Review.Ortho Res Online J. 3(5). OPROJ.000574.2018. DOI: 10.31031/OPROJ.2018.03.000574

69. University of Rochester Medical Center. (n.d.). The Biopsychosocial Approach. Retrieved from https://www.urmc.rochester.edu/medialibraries/urmcmedia/education/md/documents/biopsychosocial-model-approach.pdfhttps://www.cdc.gov/nchs/fastats/diseases-and-conditions.htm

70. Yaribeygi, H., Panahi, Y., Sahraei, H., Johnston, T. P., & Sahebkar, A. (2017). The impact of stress on body function: A review. EXCLI journal, 16, 1057-1072.https://www.merriam-webster.com/dictionary/disease

71. Chou R, Deyo R, Friedly J, et al. Nonpharmacologic Therapies for Low Back Pain. Annals of Internal Medicine. 2017;167(8):493-505. doi:10.7326/l17-0395.

72. Miller J, Gross A, Dsylva J, et al. Manual therapy and exercise for neck pain: A systematic review. Manual Therapy. 2010;15(4):334-354. doi:10.1016/j.math.2010.02.007.

73. Cheatham SW, Lee M, Cain M, et al. : The efficacy of instrument assisted soft tissue mobilization: a systematic review. J Can Chiropr Assoc, 2016, 60: 200–211.

74. ngel G. The need for a new medical model: a challenge for biomedicine. Science. 1977;196(4286):129-136. doi:10.1126/science.847460.

75. Shete K, Suryawanshi P, Gandhi N. Management of low back pain in computer users: A multidisciplinary approach. Journal of Craniovertebral Junction and Spine. 2012;3(1):7-10. doi:10.4103/0974-8237.110117.

76. Kamper SJ, Apeldoorn AT, Chiarotto A, et al. Multidisciplinary biopsychosocial rehabilitation for chronic low back pain: Cochrane systematic review and meta-analysis. Bmj. 2015;350. doi:10.1136/bmj.h444.

77. Guzmán J, Esmail R, Karjalainen K, Malmivaara A Irvin E, Bombardier C et al. Multidisciplinary rehabilitation for chronic low back pain: systematic review BMJ 2001; 322 :1511-1516. doi:10.1136/bmj.322.7301.1511.

78. Korff MRV. Long-term use of opioids for complex chronic pain. Best Practice & Research Clinical Rheumatology. 2013;27(5):663-672. doi:10.1016/j.berh.2013.09.011.

79. Machado GC, Maher CG, Ferreira PH, Day RO, Pinheiro MB, Ferreira ML. Non-steroidal anti-inflammatory drugs for spinal pain: a systematic review and meta-analysis. Annals of the Rheumatic Diseases. 2017;76(7):1269-1278. doi:10.1136/annrheumdis-2016-210597.

80. Varas-Lorenzo C, Riera-Guardia N, Calingaert B, et al. Stroke risk and NSAIDs: a systematic review of observational studies. Pharmacoepidemiology and Drug Safety. 2011;20(12):1225-1236. doi:10.1002/pds.2227.

81. Turk DC, Okifuji A. Treatment of Chronic Pain Patients: Clinical Outcomes, Cost-Effectiveness, and Cost-Benefits of Multidisciplinary Pain Centers. Critical Reviews in Physical and Rehabilitation Medicine. 1998;10(2):181-208. doi:10.1615/critrevphysrehabilmed.v10.i2.40.

82. Mavrocordatos et al. Benefits of the multidisciplinary team for the patient

83. Espejo-Antúnez L, Tejeda JF-H, Albornoz-Cabello M, et al. Dry needling in the management of myofascial trigger points: A systematic review of randomized controlled trials. Complementary Therapies in Medicine. 2017;33:46-57. doi:10.1016/j.ctim.2017.06.003.

84. Madsen MV, Gotzsche PC, Hrobjartsson A. Acupuncture treatment for pain: systematic review of randomised clinical trials with acupuncture, placebo acupuncture, and no acupuncture groups. Bmj. 2009;338. doi:10.1136/bmj.a3115.

85. Furlan, Andrea. Systematic review of acupuncture for chronic low-back pain . Japanese Acupuncture and Moxibustion, 2010; .6(1): 37-44

86. Rubinstein SM, Terwee CB, Assendelft WJ, Boer MRD, Tulder MWV. Spinal manipulative therapy for acute low-back pain. Spine. 2011;36(13):825-846. doi:10.1002/14651858.cd008880.pub2.

87. Stecco, C. (2015). Functional Atlas of the Human Fascial System. Churchill Livingstone Elsevier.

88. Stecco, L. (2016). Atlas of Physiology of the Muscular Fascia. Piccin.

89. Bordoni, B., & Zanier, E. (2015). Understanding fibroblasts in order to comprehend the osteopathic treatment of the fascia. *Evidence-Based Complementary and Alternative Medicine, 2015*. https://doi.org/10.1155/2015/860934

90. Gauglitz, G., Korting, H., Pavicic, T., Ruzicka, T., & Jeschke, M. (2011). Hypertrophic scarring and keloids: Pathomechanisms and current and emerging treatment strategies. *Molecular Medicine, 17*(1-2), 113-125. https://doi.org/10.2119/molmed.2009.00153

91. McCulloch, J., & Kloth, L. (2010). Wound Healing: Evidence-Based Management (4th ed.).

92. Bordoni, B., & Zanier, E. (2015). Anatomic connections of the diaphragm: Influence of respiration on the body system. *Journal of Multidisciplinary Healthcare, 8*, 281-291. https://doi.org/10.2147/JMDH.S70111

93. Gauglitz, G. G., Korting, H. C., Pavicic, T., Ruzicka, T., & Jeschke, M. G. (2011). Hypertrophic scarring and keloids: Pathomechanisms and current and emerging treatment strategies. *Molecular Medicine, 17*(1-2), 113-125. https://doi.org/10.2119/molmed.2009.00153

94. Kumka, M., & Bonar, J. (2012). Fascia: A morphological description and classification system based on a literature review. *Journal of the Canadian Chiropractic Association, 56*(3).

95. Benjamin, M. (2009). The fascia of the limbs and back. *Journal of Anatomy, 214*. https://doi.org/10.1111/j.1469-7580.2008.01011.x

96. Barnes, J. (1990). *Myofascial Release*. Paoli, PA: John F. Barnes, P.T. and Rehabilitation Services, Inc.

97. Yang, C., Du, Y., Wu, J., et al. (2015). Fascia and Primo Vascular System. *Evidence-Based Complementary and Alternative Medicine, 2015*, 1-6. https://doi.org/10.1155/2015/303769

98. Findley, T. W. (2011). Fascia Research from a Clinician/Scientist's Perspective. *International Journal of Therapeutic Massage and Bodywork, 4*(4), 1-6.

99. Willard, F. H., Vleeming, A., Schuenke, M. D., Danneels, L., & Schleip, R. (2012). The thoracolumbar fascia: Anatomy, function and clinical considerations. *Journal of Anatomy, 221*, 507-536. https://doi.org/10.1111/j.1469-7580.2012.01511.x

100. Litchford, M. (2012). Nutrition Focused Physical Assessment: Making Clinical Connections.

# References

101. Vasquez, A. (Date not provided). Textbook of Clinical Nutrition and Functional Medicine, Vol. 1: Essential Knowledge for Safe Action and Effective Treatment (Inflammation Mastery & Functional Inflammology).
102. Bennett, P., & Bland, J. (2010). *Textbook of Functional Medicine*.
103. Sanchez A, Reeser JL, Lau HS, Yahiku PY, Willard RE, McMillan PJ, Cho SY, Magie AR, Register UD. Role of sugars in human neutrophilic phagocytosis. Am J Clin Nutr. 1973 Nov;26(11):1180-4. doi: 10.1093/ajcn/26.11.1180. PMID: 4541857.
104. IASTM Image: https://www.temu.com/5pcs-set-stainless-steel-iastm-therapy-massage-tools-tissue-fascia-recovery-muscle-massager-guasha-scraping-gua-sha-massage-tool-g-601099540868938.html?
105. Case Studies Video Link: https://advancedsofttissuerelease.com/treatment-videos-2/
106. Hartvigsen J, Hancock MJ, Kongsted A, et al. What low back pain is and why we need to pay attention. *Lancet*. 2018;391(10137):2356-2367.
107. Engel GL. The need for a new medical model: a challenge for biomedicine. *Science*. 1977;196(4286):129-136.
108. Borrell-Carrió F, Suchman AL, Epstein RM. The biopsychosocial model 25 years later: principles, practice, and scientific inquiry. *Ann Fam Med*. 2004;2(6):576-582.
109. Brinjikji W, Luetmer PH, Comstock B, et al. MRI findings of disc degeneration are more prevalent in adults with low back pain than in asymptomatic individuals. *AJNR Am J Neuroradiol*. 2015;36(12):2394-2399.
110. Lane MM, Davis JA, Beattie S, et al. Ultra-processed food exposure and adverse health outcomes: umbrella review of epidemiological meta-analyses. *BMJ*. 2024;384:e077310.
111. Qing L, et al. Exploring the association between Dietary Inflammatory Index and chronic pain in U.S. adults. *Sci Rep*. 2024;14:58030.
112. Lis AM, Black KM, Korn H, Nordin M. Association between sitting and occupational low back pain. *Eur Spine J*. 2006;16(2):283-298.
113. Mahdavi SB, et al. Association between sedentary behavior and low back pain: a systematic review and meta-analysis. *Spine J*. 2021;21(11):1875-1888.
114. Cherkin DC, Sherman KJ, Balderson BH, et al. Effect of mindfulness-based stress reduction vs cognitive behavioral therapy or usual care on back pain and functional limitations in adults with chronic low back pain. *JAMA*. 2016;315(12):1240-1249.
115. Hayden JA, Ellis J, Ogilvie R, et al. Exercise therapy for chronic low back pain. *Cochrane Database Syst Rev*. 2021;9(9):CD009790.
116. Kamper SJ, Apeldoorn AT, Chiarotto A, et al. Multidisciplinary biopsychosocial rehabilitation for chronic low back pain: systematic review and meta-analysis. *BMJ*. 2015;350:h444.
117. Vlaeyen JWS, Linton SJ. Fear-avoidance and its consequences in chronic musculoskeletal pain: a state of the art. *Pain*. 2000;85(3):317-332.
118. den Bandt HL, Paulis WD, Beckwée D, et al. Pain mechanisms in low back pain: a systematic review and meta-analysis. *J Orthop Sports Phys Ther*. 2019;49(3):e1-e15.
119. Lewik G, et al. Postoperative epidural fibrosis: challenges and opportunities. *Int J Mol Sci*. 2023;24(24):11007250.
120. Monument MJ, et al. Neuroinflammatory mechanisms of connective tissue fibrosis. *BioMed Res Int*. 2015;2015:1-13.
121. Langevin HM, Fox JR, Koptiuch C, et al. Ultrasound evidence of altered lumbar connective tissue structure in human subjects with chronic low back pain. *BMC Musculoskelet Disord*. 2009;10:151.
122. Langevin HM, Fox JR, Koptiuch C, et al. Reduced thoracolumbar fascia shear strain in human chronic low back pain. *BMC Musculoskelet Disord*. 2011;12:203.

# References

123. Ghai B, et al. Vitamin D supplementation in patients with chronic low back pain: an open label randomized clinical trial. *Pain Physician.* 2017;20(1):E99-E105.
124. Lee TJ, et al. Updated meta-analysis reveals limited efficacy of vitamin D supplementation in chronic low back pain. *Anticancer Res.* 2024;44(??):??-??.